Malaria control
in complex emergencies

AN INTER-AGENCY
FIELD HANDBOOK

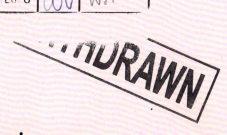
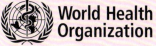
World Health Organization

WHO Library Cataloguing-in-Publication Data

Malaria control in complex emergencies : an inter-agency field handbook /
World Health Organization ... [et al.].

1. Malaria – prevention and control. 2. Emergencies. 3. Malaria –
drug therapy. 4. Refugees. 5. Disease outbreaks. 6. Mosquito control.
7. Developing countries. I. World Health Organization.

ISBN 92 4 159389 X   (NLM classification: WC 765)
                                      WHO/HTM/MAL/2005.1107

Cover photo: USAID
Designed by minimum graphics
Printed in Switzerland

Contents

Preface

Complex emergencies are characterized by insecurity and mass population movements. At the end of the year 2000, an estimated 135 million people – including refugees, returnees and internally displaced persons – were affected by complex emergencies.[1] More than 40 million people in Africa – more than 75% of them women and children – were displaced from their homes, either within their own countries or to neighbouring countries. The areas of the world whose populations are most affected by complex emergencies are often those with the greatest malaria burden. Consequently, malaria is a significant cause of death and illness in complex emergency situations.

Effective malaria control programmes prevent malaria transmission by promoting personal protection measures and effective vector control strategies, and providing appropriate case management with early diagnosis and effective treatment. However, malaria control in complex emergency situations is often difficult because of the breakdown of existing health services and programmes, displacement of health care workers and field staff with malaria expertise, movement of non-immune people to endemic areas, and concentrations of people, often already in poor health, in high-risk, high-exposure settings.

This interagency handbook was developed by the Roll Back Malaria (RBM) Technical Support Network on Complex Emergencies. It focuses on effective malaria control responses to complex emergencies, particularly during the acute phase when reliance on international humanitarian assistance is greatest. It provides policy-makers, planners, field programme managers and medical coordinators with practical guidance on designing and implementing measures to reduce malaria morbidity and mortality. Such measures must address the needs of both the displaced and the host

---

[1] Including Angola, Burundi, the Congo, the Democratic Republic of the Congo, Guinea, Liberia, Rwanda, Sierra Leone, Somalia and Sudan. This estimate does not include the refugee-affected populations in the Central African Republic or in western parts of the United Republic of Tanzania.

populations and must accommodate the changes in those needs as an acute emergency evolves into a more stable situation.

The handbook is organized as follows:

Chapter 1, Introduction – introduces complex emergencies and malaria control.

Chapter 2, Initial assessment and planning – describes how to assess the burden of malaria in an emergency and how to identify those most at risk, as well as how to use the information collected to design an effective response.

Chapter 3, Surveillance – discusses the establishment of surveillance systems to monitor the malaria situation.

Chapter 4, Outbreak preparedness and response – describes how to prepare for and respond to a sudden increase in malaria cases.

Chapter 5, Case management – provides an overview of methods of diagnosis, treatment and patient care in complex emergencies.

Chapter 6, Prevention – describes the most useful approaches and tools currently available for vector control and personal protection from malaria in complex emergencies.

Chapter 7, Community participation and health education – discusses how to mobilize affected communities to participate in malaria control interventions.

Chapter 8, Research and evaluation – focuses on evaluating the effectiveness of prevention and treatment measures, and identifies priority operational research issues for malaria control in complex emergencies.

In addition, a glossary is provided at the beginning of the handbook. Suggestions for further reading are included at the end of several chapters.

Ideal – or "gold standard" – approaches to malaria control may not always be feasible in complex emergencies, and interventions will need to be adapted to the realities of each situation. Using this handbook, however, humanitarian agencies should be able to implement effective and concerted responses to the malaria problems.

As new information becomes available, updates to the handbook will be published. Comments and suggestions are most welcome and should be sent to RBM/Complex Emergencies at WHO (E-mail: rbmemergencies@who.int).

Contributors

This handbook is an initiative of the Roll Back Malaria Technical Support Network on Complex Emergencies. In 1998, when development of the handbook began, the RBM Network, facilitated by WHO, brought together the following agencies involved in malaria control in complex emergencies:

Basic Support for Institutionalizing Child Survival (BASICS), USA
Centers for Disease Control and Prevention (CDC), USA
Mailman School of Public Health, Columbia University, USA
Epicentre, France
HealthNet International, Netherlands
International Committee of the Red Cross, Switzerland
International Federation of Red Cross and Red Crescent Societies, Switzerland
International Organization for Migration, Switzerland
Karolinska Institute, Sweden
London School of Hygiene & Tropical Medicine, England
Malaria Consortium, England
Médecins du Monde, France
Médecins Sans Frontières (MSF), France
MSF Belgium
MSF Holland
Menzies School of Public Health, Charles Darwin University, Australia
Merlin, England
Ministry of Health, Angola
Ministry of Health, Liberia
Office of the United Nations High Commissioner for Refugees, Switzerland
United Nations Children's Fund (UNICEF), USA
UNICEF, Kenya
Wellcome Trust – Shoklo Malaria Research Unit, Thailand

WHO:
  Headquarters, Geneva
  Regional Office for Africa (AFRO)
  Regional Office for Europe (EURO)
  Regional Office for South-East Asia (SEARO)
  Regional Office for the Eastern Mediterranean (EMRO)
  Regional Office for Western Pacific (WPRO)
  WHO Afghanistan
  WHO Angola
  WHO Kenya
  WHO Liaison Office for South Sudan (Nairobi)

The original draft of this document was produced by a writing committee from the RBM Technical Support Network on Complex Emergencies, consisting of:

Richard Allan (Merlin)
Kathy Attawell (Malaria Consortium, editorial consultant)
Suna Balkan (MSF France, Chapters 3 and 4)
Peter Bloland (CDC Atlanta, Chapter 5)
Kabir Cham (WHO Geneva)
Maire Connolly (WHO Geneva)
Charles Delacollette (WHO Geneva, Chapter 2)
Marc Gastellu (MSF France, Chapters 3 and 4)
Serge Male (UNHCR Geneva)
Sylvia Meek (Malaria Consortium UK, Chapter 6)
François Nosten (Shoklo Malaria Research Unit, Thailand, Chapter 5)
Aafje Rietveld (WHO Geneva)
Mark Rowland (HealthNet International, Chapters 6 and 8)
Catherine Surrell (MSF France, Chapter 3)
Holly Williams (CDC Atlanta, Chapter 7)

The World Health Organization Roll Back Malaria department, with the assistance of the Malaria Consortium, was responsible for the final technical review.

The final manuscript was edited by Sarah Ballance.

Acknowledgements

The writing committee and agencies who compiled this handbook grate-fully acknowledge all the colleagues who have reviewed chapters before publication, particularly the following field and academic specialists who contributed to the further development and reviews of the text:

Guy Barnish (Liverpool School of Tropical Medicine), Harini Boteju (Malaria Consortium), Kate Burns (UNHCR), Jane Crawley (WHO), Linda Doull (Merlin), Nadine Ezard (WHO), Pierre Guillet (WHO), Christa Hook (MSF UK), Stéphane Hugonnet (MSF Switzerland), Isabelle Lessard (WHO), John MacArthur (CDC), Peter Maes (MSF Belgium), David Nabarro (WHO), Bernard Nahlen (WHO), Robin Nandy (International Rescue Committee), Jose Nkuni (WHO), Pierro Olliaro (WHO), Peter Olumese (WHO), William Perea (Epicentre), Jean Rigal (MSF France), Pascal Ringwald (WHO), Allan Schapira (WHO), Robert Scherpbier (WHO), Murtada Sesay (WHO), Bob Taylor (WHO), Awash Teklehaimanot (WHO), Michel Thuriaux (WHO), Peter Trigg (WHO), Michel van Herp (MSF Belgium), Hans Veeken (MSF Holland), Martin Weber (WHO), Jacob Williams (WHO).

Thanks are also due to the nongovernmental organizations, United Nations agencies, and operational field partners of RBM for their support.

Finally, we thank UNHCR, the United Kingdom Department for International Development, the US Department of State Bureau of Population, Refugees and Migration, and WHO for generous financial support for this publication.

Acronyms and abbreviations

ACT	artemisinin-based combination therapy
CDC	Centers for Disease Control and Prevention
CMR	crude mortality rate
CSF	cerebrospinal fluid
DFID	Department for International Development (United Kingdom)
DRC	Democratic Republic of the Congo
GPS	global positioning system
IDP	internally displaced person
IFRC	International Federation of Red Cross and Red Crescent Societies
IM	intramuscular
IMCI	Integrated Management of Childhood Illness
IRC	International Rescue Committee
IRS	indoor residual spraying
ITM	insecticide-treated material
ITN	insecticide-treated net
ITP	intermittent preventive treatment
IV	intravenous
LP	lumbar puncture
MOH	ministry of health
MSF	Médecins Sans Frontières
NG	nasogastric
NGO	nongovernmental organization
NMCP	national malaria control programme
ORS	oral rehydration solution
PVO	private voluntary organization
RBM	Roll Back Malaria
RDT	rapid diagnostic test
SP	sulfadoxine–pyrimethamine
UNDHA	United Nations Department for Humanitarian Affairs
UNDMT	United Nations Disaster Management Teams
UNDP	United Nations Development Programme
UNICEF	United Nations Children's Fund
UNHCR	Office of the United Nations High Commissioner for Refugees
USAID	United States Agency for International Development
WFP	World Food Programme
WHO	World Health Organization

Glossary

The definitions given below apply to the terms as used in this handbook. They may have different meanings in other contexts.

A

acute emergency phase Begins immediately after the impact of the disaster and may last for up to 3 months. Characterized by initial chaos and a high crude mortality rate (CMR). Ends when daily CMR drops below 1/10 000 people.

adherence (compliance) Health-related behaviour that abides by the recommendations of a doctor or other health care provider or of an investigator in a research project.

agranulocytosis Severe deficiency of certain white blood cells as a result of damage to the bone marrow by toxic drugs or chemicals.

anaemia A reduction in the quantity of the oxygen-carrying pigment haemoglobin in the blood. The main symptoms are tiredness, breathlessness on exertion, pallor and poor resistance to infection.

Anopheles A genus of widely distributed mosquitoes, occurring in tropical and temperate regions and containing some 400 species. Malaria parasites (*Plasmodium*) are transmitted to humans through the bite of female *Anopheles* mosquitoes.

Anopheles, infected Female *Anopheles* with oocysts of malaria parasites on the midgut wall (with or without sporozoites in the salivary glands).

Anopheles, infective Female *Anopheles* with sporozoites in the salivary glands (with or without oocysts in the midgut).

antipyretic A drug that reduces fever by lowering the body temperature.

anthropophilic Descriptive of mosquitoes that show a preference for feeding on humans even when non-human hosts are available. A relative term requiring quantification to indicate the extent of the preference.

asymptomatic Not showing any symptoms of disease, whether disease is present or not. (See **parasitaemia** for "asymptomatic malaria".)

attack rate The cumulative incidence of infection in a group observed over a period during an epidemic.

auscultation Listening, usually with the aid of a stethoscope, to the sounds produced by the movement of gas/air or fluid within the body, to diagnose abnormalities, for example in the lungs.

B

bacteraemia Presence of bacteria in the blood.

bias Any trend in the collection, analysis, interpretation, publication or review of data that can lead to conclusions that are systematically different from the truth.

blood meal Ingestion by a female mosquito of blood obtained from a vertebrate host; also, the ingested blood.

bradycardia Slowing of the heart rate to less than 50 beats per minute.

breeding site (place) Site where eggs, larvae or pupae of mosquitoes are found; larval habitat.

C

case A person who has the particular disease, health disorder or condition that meets the case definition.

case definition A set of diagnostic criteria that must be fulfilled for an individual to be regarded as a "case" of a particular disease for surveillance and outbreak investigation purposes. Case definitions can be based on clinical criteria, laboratory criteria or a combination of the two.

case-fatality rate The proportion of cases of a specified condition that are fatal within a specified time (usually expressed as a percentage).

census Enumeration of a population. A census usually records the identities of all persons in every place of residence, with age or date of birth, sex, occupation, national origin, language, marital status, income, and relationship to head of household, in addition to information on the dwelling place.

chemoprophylaxis Administration of a chemical to prevent either the development of an infection or the progression of an infection to active manifest disease.

cluster sampling A sampling method in which each selected unit is a group of people (e.g. all persons in a city block, a family) rather than an individual.

community health worker (CHW) A member of the community who is integrated into primary health care programmes after a short training on health-related issues, and who acts as intermediary between the community and the health services. CHWs may be paid staff or volunteers (CHVs).

compliance See **adherence**.

confidence interval A computed interval with a given probability (e.g. 95%) that the true value of a variable (e.g. a mean, proportion or rate) is contained within that interval.

conjunctival Relating to the conjunctiva, the thin mucosa covering the inside of the eyelids and the sclera (the white part of the eye).

contact (of an infection) A person or animal that has been in such association with an infected person or animal or a contaminated environment as to have had opportunity to acquire the infection.

coverage A measure of the extent to which services cover the potential need for these services in a community. It is expressed as a proportion in which the numerator is the number of services rendered and the denominator is the number of instances in which the service should have been rendered.

cross-sectional study (disease frequency survey; prevalence study) A study that examines the relationship between diseases (or other health-related characteristics) and other variables of interest as they exist in a defined population at one particular time. The presence or absence of disease and the presence or absence (or, if they are quantitative, the level) of the other variables are determined in each member of the study population or in a representative sample at one particular time. The relationship between a variable and the disease can be examined in terms both of the prevalence of disease in different population subgroups defined according to the presence or absence (or level) of the variables and of the presence or absence (or level) of the variables in the diseased versus the non-diseased. A cross-sectional study usually records disease prevalence rather than incidence and cannot necessarily determine cause-and-effect relationships.

D

demography The study of populations, especially with reference to size and density, fertility, mortality, growth, age distribution, migration and vital statistics, and the interaction of all these with social and economic conditions.

district hospital A hospital with the capacity to manage first-referral cases but with medical services usually limited to emergency obstetrical and surgical care and follow-up, and inpatient and rehabilitative care. In principle, facilities include laboratory, blood bank, and X-ray services.

E

effectiveness A measure of the extent to which a specific intervention, procedure, regimen or service, when deployed in the field in routine circumstances, does what it is intended to do for a specified population; a measure of the extent to which a health care intervention fulfils its objectives.

efficacy The extent to which a specific intervention, procedure, regimen or service produces a beneficial result under ideal conditions; the benefit or utility to the individual or population of the service, treatment regimen or intervention. Ideally, determination of efficacy is based on the results of a randomized controlled trial.

efficiency The effects or end results achieved in relation to the effort expended in terms of money, resources and time; the extent to which the resources used to provide a specific intervention, procedure, regimen or service of known efficacy and effectiveness are minimized; a measure of the economy (or cost in resources) with which a procedure of known efficacy and effectiveness is carried out; the process of making the best use of scarce resources.

endemic Description applied to malaria when there is a constant measurable incidence both of cases and of natural transmission in an area over a succession of years.

endophagy Tendency of mosquitoes to feed indoors.

endophily Tendency of mosquitoes to rest indoors.

epidemic Description applied to malaria when the incidence of cases (other than seasonal increases) in an area rises rapidly and markedly above its usual level or when the infection occurs in an area where it was not previously present.

epidemic curve A graphic plotting of the distribution of cases by time of onset.

epidemiology The study of the distribution and determinants of health-related conditions or events in specified populations, and the application of this study to the control of health problems.

essential drugs Therapeutic substances that are indispensable for rational care of the majority of diseases in a given population.

evaluation A process that attempts to determine as systematically and objectively as possible the relevance, effectiveness and impact of activities in relation to their objectives.

exophagy Tendency of mosquitoes to feed outdoors.

exophily Tendency of mosquitoes to rest outdoors.

F

focus group Small convenience sample of people brought together to discuss a topic or issue with the aim of ascertaining the range and intensity of their views, rather than arriving at a consensus. Focus groups are used, for example, to appraise perceptions of health problems, assess the acceptability of a field study or refine the questions to be used in a field study.

G

gamete Mature sexual form, male or female. In malaria parasites, the female gametes (macrogametes) and the male gametes (microgametes) normally develop in the mosquito.

gametocytes Parent cell of a gamete. In malaria parasites, the female and male gametocytes develop in the red blood cell. Very young gametocytes cannot usually be distinguished from trophozoites.

H

haemoglobinuria The presence of haemoglobin in the urine

haemolysis The destruction of red blood cells.

health care system The organization of health care services within a designated geographical area (e.g. country, province, district, camp).

hepatic Relating to the liver.

host A person or other living animal, including birds and arthropods, harbouring or providing subsistence to a parasite. In an epidemiological context, the host may be the population or group; biological, social and behavioural characteristics of this group that are relevant to health are called "host factors".

host, definitive In parasitology, the host in which sexual maturation occurs. In malaria, the definitive host is the mosquito (invertebrate host).

host, intermediate In parasitology, the host in which asexual forms of the parasite develop. In malaria, the intermediate host is a human or other mammal or bird (vertebrate host).

household One or more persons who occupy a dwelling; may or may not be a family. The term is also used to describe the dwelling unit in which the persons live.

hypersensitivity Responding exaggeratedly to the presence of a particular antigen.

I

immunity, acquired Resistance acquired by a host as a result of previous exposure to a natural pathogen or substance that is foreign to the host.

incidence The number of instances of illness commencing, or of persons falling ill, during a given period in a specified population.

incidence rate The rate at which new events occur in a population. The numerator is the number of new events that occur in a defined period and the denominator is the population at risk of experiencing these events during this period, sometimes expressed as person-time.

indicator A measure that shows whether a standard has been reached. It is used to assess and communicate the results of programmes as well as the process or methods used. Indicators can be qualitative or quantitative.

infection, mixed Malaria infection with more than one species of *Plasmodium*.

informed consent Voluntary consent given by a subject (i.e. person or a responsible proxy such as a parent) for participation in a study, immunization programme, treatment regimen, etc., after being informed of the purpose, methods, procedures, benefits and risks, and, when relevant, the degree of uncertainty about outcomes. The essential criteria of informed consent are that the subject has both knowledge and comprehension, that consent is freely given without duress or undue influence, and that the right of withdrawal at any time is clearly communicated to the subject.

inpatient facility A health care institution that provides lodging, nursing and continuous medical care for patients within a facility and with an organized professional staff.

K

knowledge, attitudes, practice (KAP) survey A formal survey, using face-to-face interviews, in which people are asked standardized pre-tested questions dealing with their knowledge, attitudes and practice concerning a given health or health-related problem.

knockdown Rapid immobilization of an insect by an insecticide, without necessarily causing early death.

L

larva The pre-adult or immature stage hatching from a mosquito egg.

loading dose An initial higher dose of a drug, given with the objective of rapidly providing an effective drug concentration.

logistics The procurement, maintenance and transport of material, personnel and facilities; management of the details of an undertaking.

M

merozoite A stage in the life cycle of the malaria parasite. Product of segmentation of a tissue schizont, or of an erythrocytic schizont before entering a new host cell. Merozoites are found either separated from or contained in the original schizont.

mesoendemicity A pattern of malaria transmission typically found among small rural communities in subtropical zones, with varying intensity of transmission depending on local circumstances.

mobile clinic See **outreach clinic.**

monitoring Episodic measurement of the effect of an intervention on the health status of a population or environment; not to be confused with surveillance, although surveillance techniques may be used in monitoring. The process of collecting and analysing information about the implementation of a programme for the purpose of identifying problems, such as non-compliance, and taking corrective action. In management: the episodic review of the implementation of an activity, seeking to ensure that inputs, deliveries, work schedules, targeted outputs and other required actions are proceeding according to plan.

morbidity Any departure, subjective or objective, from a state of physiological or psychological well-being. *Sickness*, *illness*, and *morbid condition* are similarly defined and synonymous. Morbidity can be measured as: (a) persons who are ill; (b) the illnesses experienced by these persons; and (c) the duration of these illnesses.

mortality rate An estimate of the proportion of a population dying during a specified period. The numerator is the number of persons dying during the period and the denominator is the total number of the population, usually estimated as the mid-year population.

myalgia Pain in the muscles.

N

needs assessment A systematic procedure for determining the nature and extent of problems that directly or indirectly affect the health of a specified population. Needs assessment makes use of epidemiological, socio-demographic and qualitative methods to describe health problems and their environmental, social, economic and behavioural determinants. The aim is to identify unmet health care needs and make recommendations about ways to address these needs.

O

oedema Swelling caused by an excess of fluid in the tissues.

oliguria The production of an abnormally small amount of urine over a period of time.

outpatient clinic A facility for diagnosis, treatment and care of ambulatory patients.

outreach (clinic, team) The extending of services or assistance beyond fixed facilities.

P

pallor Paleness.

palmar Relating to the palms of the hands.

parasitaemia Condition in which malaria parasites are present in the blood. If this condition in the human subject is not accompanied by fever or other symptoms of malaria except for a possible enlargement of the spleen, it is known as asymptomatic parasitaemia, and the person exhibiting the condition is known as an asymptomatic parasite carrier.

parenteral Relates to drug administration by any route other than oral, e.g. by injection.

paroxysms Cyclic manifestation of acute illness in malaria characterized by a rise in temperature with accompanying symptoms; usually caused by invasion of the blood by a brood of erythrocytic parasites.

Plasmodium Genus of parasites causing human malaria (*Plasmodium falciparum*, *P. vivax*, *P. ovale*, *P. malariae*).

population structure Composition of the population, usually by age and sex.

preparedness Readiness to prevent, mitigate, respond to and cope with the effects of a disaster or epidemic.

prevalence The number of instances of a given disease or other condition in a given population at a designated time, with no distinction between new and old cases. Prevalence may be recorded at a specific moment (point prevalence) or over a given period of time (period prevalence).

prevalence rate The total number of all individuals who have a disease or condition at a particular time (or during a particular period) divided by the population at risk of having the attribute or disease at that point in time or midway through that period.

prevention Actions aimed at eradicating, eliminating or minimizing the impact of disease and disability or, if none of these is feasible, retarding the progress of disease and disability. The concept of prevention is best defined in the context of levels, called primary, secondary, and tertiary prevention. In epidemiological terms, primary prevention aims to reduce the incidence of disease; secondary prevention aims to reduce the prevalence of disease by shortening its duration; and tertiary prevention aims to reduce the number and/or impact of complications.

proportion See under **ratio**.

pulmonary Relating to, associated with or affecting the lungs.

R

random sample A sample that is arrived at by selecting sample units in such a way that each possible unit has a fixed and determinate probability of selection. Random allocation follows a predetermined plan that is usually devised with the aid of a table of random numbers. Random sampling should not be confused with haphazard assignment.

rate A measure of the frequency of occurrence of a phenomenon. In epidemiology, demography and vital statistics, a rate is an expression of the frequency with which an event occurs in a defined population in a specified period of time. The use of rates rather than raw numbers is essential for comparison of experience between populations at different times, different places, or among different groups of persons. The components of a rate are the numerator, the denominator, the specified time in which events occur, and usually a multiplier, a power of 10, that converts the rate from an awkward fraction or decimal to a whole number.

$$\text{rate} = \frac{\text{number of events in specified period}}{\text{average population during the period}} \times 10^n$$

ratio The value obtained by dividing one quantity by another; a general term of which rate, proportion, percentage, etc. are sub-sets. The important difference between a proportion and a ratio is that the numerator of a proportion is included in the population defined by the denominator, whereas this is not necessarily so for a ratio. A ratio is an expression of the relationship between a numerator and a denominator where the two are usually separate and distinct quantities, neither being included in the other.

recrudescence Repeated manifestation of an infection after a period of latency following the primary attack. It is used particularly in the context of treatment failure of *Plasmodium falciparum*, and is often the result of non-adherence to the treatment regimen, especially with short-acting drugs such as quinine and the artemisinins.

relapse Renewed manifestation (of clinical symptoms and/or parasitaemia) of malaria infection separated from previous manifestations of the same infection by an interval greater than that related to the normal periodicity of the paroxysms. The term is used mainly for renewed manifestation due to survival of exo-erythrocytic forms of *Plasmodium vivax* or *P. ovale*.

reservoir (of infection) Any person, animal, arthropod, plant, soil or substance, or a combination of these, in which an infectious agent normally lives and multiplies, on which it depends primarily for survival, and where it reproduces itself in such a manner that it can be transmitted to a susceptible host. The natural habitat of the infectious agent.

resistance Ability of a parasite strain to multiply or to survive in the presence of concentrations of a drug that normally destroy parasites of the same species or prevent their multiplication. Ability in a population of insects to tolerate doses of an insecticide that would prove lethal to the majority of individuals in a normal population of the same species; developed as a result of selection pressure by the insecticide.

retention (in ITN programme) An indicator used to establish whether nets remain with the individuals to whom they were originally distributed. Retention alone is not an indicator of the correct use of the nets.

risk The probability that an event will occur, e.g. that an individual will become ill or die within a stated period of time or by a certain age. Also a non-technical term encompassing a variety of measures of the probability of a (generally) unfavourable outcome.

S

sample A selected sub-set of a population. A sample may be random or non-random and may be representative or non-representative.

sampling The process of selecting a number of subjects from all the subjects in a particular group, or "universe". Conclusions based on sample results may be attributed only to the population from which the sample was taken. Any extrapolation to a larger or different population is a judgement or a guess and is not part of statistical inference.

schizont Intracellular asexual form of the malaria parasite, developing either in tissue or in blood cells.

sensitivity (of a screening test) The proportion of truly diseased persons in the screened population who are identified as diseased by the screening test. Sensitivity is a measure of the probability of correctly diagnosing a case, or the probability that any given case will be identified by the test. See also **specificity**.

species Group of organisms capable of exchanging genetic material with one another and incapable, by reason of their genetic constitution, of exchanging such material with any other group of organisms.

specificity (of a screening test) The proportion of truly non-diseased persons who are so identified by the screening test. Specificity is a measure of the probability of correctly identifying a non-diseased person with a screening test.

spleen rate A term used in malaria epidemiology to define the frequency of enlarged spleens detected on survey of a population in which malaria is prevalent.

splenomegaly Enlargement of the spleen.

sporozoite The infective form of the malaria parasite occurring in a mature oocyst before its rupture and in the salivary glands of the mosquito.

surveillance The process of systematic collection, orderly consolidation and evaluation of pertinent data with prompt dissemination of the results to those who need to know, particularly those who are in a position to take action.

survey An investigation in which information is systematically collected; usually carried out in a sample of a defined population group, within a defined time period. Unlike surveillance a survey is not continuous; however, if repeated regularly, surveys can form the basis of a surveillance system.

systematic sampling The procedure of selecting according to some simple, systematic rule, such as all persons whose names begin with specified alphabetical letters, who are born on certain dates, or who are located at specified points on a master list. A systematic sample may lead to errors that invalidate generalizations. For example, people's names more often begin with certain letters of the alphabet than with other letters. A systematic alphabetical sample is therefore likely to be biased.

T

target population The group of people for whom an intervention is intended.

transmission Any mechanism by which an infectious agent is spread from a source or reservoir to another person.

transmission, perennial Transmission occurring throughout the year without great variation of intensity.

transmission, seasonal Natural transmission that occurs only during some months and is totally interrupted during other months.

trend A long-term movement in an ordered series, e.g. a time series. An essential feature is movement consistently in the same direction over the long term.

triage The process of selecting for care or treatment those of highest priority or, when resources are limited, those thought most likely to benefit.

trophozoite Strictly, any asexual and growing parasite with an undivided nucleus. In malaria terminology, generally used to indicate intracellular erythrocytic forms in their early stages of development. Trophozoites may be in either a ring stage or an early amoeboid or solid stage, but always have the nucleus still undivided.

V

vector Any insect or living carrier that transports an infectious agent from an infected individual or his/her wastes to a susceptible individual or his/her food or immediate surroundings. The organism may or may not pass though a developmental cycle within the vector.

vector control Measures of any kind directed against a vector of disease and intended to limit its ability to transmit the disease.

verbal autopsy A procedure for gathering systematic information that enables the cause of death to be determined in situations where the deceased has not been medically attended. It is based on the assumption that most common and important causes of death have distinct symptom complexes that can be recognized, remembered and reported by lay respondents.

vulnerability Defencelessness, insecurity, exposure to risks, shock, and stress, and having difficulty coping with them. The potential that when something destructive happens or goes wrong, people will not be able to handle the consequences by themselves and the ability to sustain life is endangered.

Z

zoophilic Descriptive of mosquitoes showing a relative preference for non-human blood even when human hosts are readily available.

The foregoing definitions have been adapted from the following sources:

Concise medical dictionary, 5th ed (1998). Oxford, Oxford University Press.

Last J (2001). *A dictionary of epidemiology*, 4th ed. Oxford, Oxford University Press.

Slee V et al. (1996). *Health care terms*, 3rd ed. St Paul, MN, Tringa Press.

Terminology of malaria and of malaria eradication (1963). Geneva, World Health Organization.

CHAPTER 1

Introduction

This chapter:
- explains what is meant by a complex emergency and the different phases of an emergency
- discusses the impact of complex emergencies, explaining who is affected
- provides basic information about malaria parasites, malaria transmission and populations at risk, and why malaria is significant in emergency situations
- sets out the key steps of an effective emergency response.

Complex emergencies

Definition and causes

A complex emergency is a situation that affects large civilian populations with war or civil strife, food shortages and population displacement, resulting in excess mortality and morbidity.

Complex emergencies can have multiple causes, requiring responses specifically designed for the needs of those affected. Most complex emergencies follow disasters of human cause – for example, war between states, internal conflict, political persecution of ethnic groups. These situations may cause large-scale population displacement or, commonly leave communities stranded and isolated in their own homes unable to access assistance. These settings are often characterized by breakdown of social and physical infrastructure, including health care systems. They can be of sudden onset – for example, Rwanda in 1994 or East Timor (now Timor-Leste) in 1999 – or may develop more slowly – for example, Afghanistan and Sudan. In many emergencies, both natural and human factors play a role and their interaction can exacerbate the situation. For instance, drought and heavy rains exacerbated existing complex emergency situations in Burundi, the Democratic Republic of the Congo (DRC), north-eastern Kenya, and Somalia. Manipulation of access to food supplies, water or agricultural land can create famine situations in specific communities as happened, for example, in southern Sudan, or even displace entire populations.

Different phases of complex emergencies

Complex emergencies are not stable, and the situation can change rapidly and unpredictably. Thus there are many different descriptions of the various phases of an emergency. Box 1.1 presents a summary version that may be useful, and Box 1.2 describes key characteristics of the acute phase. Most complex emergencies continue to shift between different phases for many years, until the causes of the original conflict are resolved and order is restored.

Box 1.1 **The main phases of emergencies**

Acute phase	Immediate: 0–4 weeks
	Stabilization: 4–10 weeks
Chronic phase	Recovery: several months
	Settlement or repatriation: months or years

Box 1.2 **Characteristics of the acute phase of emergencies**

- Mortality rates are usually high (over 1/10 000 population per day).
- Access for the affected population to effective health care is poor (the health infrastructure may be overwhelmed, inadequate or non-existent).
- Appropriate response is beyond local or national capacity.
- Normal coordination mechanisms may have broken down.

Mortality rates may remain high long after the acute phase is over, particularly when there is ongoing conflict. For example, rates have remained high in war-affected communities in eastern DRC since 1998.

The impact of complex emergencies

It is important to understand how people are affected during different phases of emergencies, and to be aware that complex emergencies have an impact on resident or host populations as well as refugee and internally displaced populations. The emergency response must be adapted to the needs of different populations, as they change over time.

Impact on displaced populations

Populations affected by complex emergencies may be driven from their homes to another part of their own country to become internally displaced people (IDPs) or to a neighbouring country to become refugees. During flight and the acute phase of an emergency, these populations are particularly vulnerable to malnutrition and disease.

Camps for refugees and IDPs planned as "temporary" settlement areas during the acute phase of an emergency may ultimately become relatively stable communities. When displaced populations cannot return to their own homes or their own country for many years, camps may become long-term settlements. Examples are the Congolese and Burundian refugee camps in the United Republic of Tanzania and the Karen refugee camps in Thailand.

Refugees and IDPs who are scattered among host communities, living with host households, are a common feature of many complex situations. Often, such displaced people are not registered by national or United Nations authorities and may not receive assistance in the same way as those living in official camps or settlements. Consequently, because they have no access to basic health care, food distribution or other services, they may be particularly vulnerable. Access to displaced people scattered among host households is a challenge for emergency actors.

Impact on resident or host populations

Resident or host populations may not be directly affected by the causes of a complex emergency but can be severely affected by the effects of that emergency. Hosting large numbers of refugees or IDPs can stretch limited local resources and have a detrimental effect on the local economy. Resident populations may also be directly affected by the causes of the emergency. If conflict, political oppression or deployment of antipersonnel mines severely restricts people's movement, the resident population may be unable to access essential materials and services, such as food, land, firewood, water and health care, and may be effectively prevented from carrying out their normal employment. Conditions for the resident population may deteriorate and result in high rates of malnutrition and disease.

Sometimes the bulk of humanitarian assistance is delivered to the displaced population, who consequently have better access to essential services than the local population. This can create tension between the displaced and resident populations. The emergency response must therefore be designed to meet the needs of all populations affected by a complex emergency – refugee, IDP and resident.

Mortality and morbidity rates

Complex emergencies result in high rates of death and illness, especially during the acute phase. Crude mortality rates (see Table 1.1) are commonly used to express the severity of emergencies.

Death and illness do not affect everyone equally. Certain population groups, such as young children, are more vulnerable to the effects of malnutrition and disease. Thus, while crude mortality rates provide information about overall mortality rates in a population, they do not help to identify the groups most at risk. In complex emergencies, initial assessment and ongoing surveillance must ensure that the most vulnerable groups are identified and that their needs are met.

Over the past decade, the majority of complex emergencies have occurred in African countries. In most instances only a small proportion of total deaths have been directly related to war trauma; most have been caused by diarrhoeal diseases, malaria, pneumonia, measles and malnutrition, all of which are preventable.

Table 1.1 **Crude mortality rates in emergencies**

Crude mortality rate (deaths/10 000 population per day)	Severity of emergency
Up to 0.5	[Normal – non-emergency]
<1	Under control
>1	Very serious
>2	Out of control
>5	Catastrophic

Malaria

Malaria is a common and life-threatening disease in many tropical and subtropical areas. It is currently endemic in over 100 countries. Each year an estimated 300 million people fall ill with malaria, and there are more than 1 million deaths. Malaria is caused by the protozoan parasite *Plasmodium* and transmitted by female *Anopheles* mosquitoes, which bite mainly between sunset and sunrise.

Parasites

Four species of malaria parasites infect people – *Plasmodium falciparum, P. vivax, P. malariae,* and *P. ovale* – of which *P. falciparum* and *P. vivax* are the most common. Falciparum malaria can be fatal, and is a priority during the acute phase of an emergency. Severe falciparum malaria has a case-fatality rate of around 10% in reasonably well-equipped hospitals.

4

Vivax malaria is an acute but not life-threatening illness associated with anaemia and splenomegaly, and causes low birth weight. Unlike *P. falciparum*, the liver stages of *P. vivax* can give rise to relapse. Malaria caused by the other *Plasmodium* species is less severe than falciparum malaria and is rarely life-threatening.

The current distribution of malaria in the world is shown in Figure 1.1.

The four human malaria species are not evenly distributed across the malaria-affected areas of the world and their relative importance varies between and within different regions. The risk of contracting malaria is therefore highly variable from country to country and even between areas in a country. *P. falciparum* is the commonest species throughout the tropics and subtropics, and predominates in sub-Saharan Africa. *P. vivax* has the widest geographical range, is present in many temperate zones but also in the subtropics, and coexists with *P. falciparum* in the Horn of Africa and in tropical parts of the Americas and Asia. *P. ovale* occurs in Africa and sporadically in south-east Asia and the western Pacific. *P. malariae* has a similar geographical distribution to *P. falciparum* but is far less common and its incidence is patchy.

It is important to know which species are present in any particular area and the relative importance of each species, because this will affect the choice of treatment. In Afghanistan, for example, 85% of malaria is caused

Figure 1.1 **Global malaria distribution in 2004**

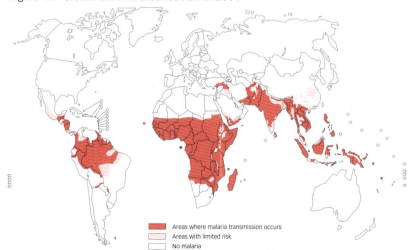

Areas where malaria transmission occurs
Areas with limited risk
No malaria

This map is a visual aid only, it is not a definitive source of information about malaria endemicity. Source: ©WHO, 2004

_ax_ and up to 15% by _P. falciparum_; in DRC, 95% of malaria is
. _falciparum_, with _P. malariae_ and _P. ovale_ accounting for the re-
5%; in Timor-Leste, 60% is caused by _P. falciparum_ and 40% by
. The relative importance of vivax and falciparum in a country may
er time. In areas of significantly mixed malaria infection, such as
Leste, it is even more important that patients with suspected malaria
be diagnosed by laboratory methods so that appropriate treatment
given for the species causing the disease. However, if microscopy
l diagnostic tests (RDTs) are not available, all cases of suspected
must be assumed to be of mixed infection and treated for both
Generally, _P. vivax_ can be treated with the same antimalarials as
barum, with the exception of sulfadoxine–pyrimethamine (SP). In
pecific circumstances, _P. vivax_ may require additional anti-relapse
ent with primaquine.

S

are about 400 different species of _Anopheles_ mosquitoes throughout
rld, but only some 60 of these are vectors of malaria under natural
ons, and only 30 are vectors of major importance. Each species has
rent behaviour pattern. Several species of _Anopheles_ can be found
st malarial areas, and different species occur in different parts of
rld. Highly efficient species, such as _A. gambiae_, _A. arabiensis_ and
estus, predominate in sub-Saharan Africa, while less efficient vec-
uch as _A. stephensi_ and _A. minimus_, predominate in Asian countries.
_us_ is an efficient vector in the forests of south-east Asia.

nicity, transmission and disease patterns (populations at risk)
ledge of the epidemiology of malaria in the area affected by an emer-
is essential, to allow appropriate prevention and case-management
gies to be planned.
e epidemiology varies by region, determining levels of immunity and
f severe disease. In highly endemic areas, people gradually develop
tial immunity to the disease, and it is therefore young children who
ost at risk from severe infection with malaria. In these areas, malaria
egnancy causes maternal anaemia, as well as spontaneous abortions,
rths and low birth weight, particularly during first and second preg-
es and in HIV-infected women. In lowland and rural areas of Africa,
ria endemicity may be very high, with perennial (where there is rain-
or more than 8 months a year) or seasonal transmission.

In areas of intense malaria transmission, such as Liberia and Sierra Leone, the population is semi-immune after childhood. Incidence of symptomatic disease remains fairly constant all year round. People in these areas may carry malaria parasites in their blood without showing clinical symptoms of disease; thus the presence of parasites in a patient's blood is not a clear indicator that malaria is the cause of the illness. While more than 60% of the population is parasite-positive at any time, young children are at increased risk of developing severe malaria in the rainy season.

Hilly, forested areas of south-east Asia also have high transmission, but severe disease is common in adults whose work obliges them to stay overnight in forests. In parts of Asia and the Americas where transmission is low to moderate, seasonal and epidemic peaks of malaria incidence are seen. In high-altitude and desert-fringe areas and in city centres malaria endemicity is usually low, with less than 10% of the population infected (although there is some transmission in cities of Africa and south Asia). In areas of unstable malaria transmission, such as the highlands of Angola, Burundi, Ethiopia, Kenya, Rwanda, Uganda and the United Republic of Tanzania and the semi-arid and desert fringes of countries in the Horn of Africa and the Sahel, the whole population may have low levels of immunity and outbreaks of malaria may affect all age and population groups. The presence of parasites in a patient's blood indicates that malaria is highly likely to be the cause of the presenting illness.

Malaria may re-emerge in areas where it was once well controlled, such as central Asian countries since the break-up of the former Soviet Union. For instance, population displacement from malaria-endemic areas of Afghanistan has contributed to the re-emergence of *P. falciparum* malaria in Tajikistan.

Recognizing malaria

Malaria is an acute febrile illness with an incubation period of 7 days or longer. Thus, a febrile illness developing less than one week after the first possible exposure is not malaria.

The most severe form is caused by *P. falciparum*, in which variable clinical features include fever, chills, headache, muscular aching and weakness, vomiting, cough, diarrhoea and abdominal pain; other symptoms related to organ failure may supervene, such as acute renal failure, generalized convulsions, and circulatory collapse, followed by coma and death. It is estimated that about 1% of patients with *P. falciparum* infection die of the disease. In complex emergencies in areas of high transmission, malaria may

7

account for up to 50% of all deaths. Prevention of progression to severe malaria disease and death depends on accurate diagnosis and prompt treatment. An effective and usable case definition for malaria is critical. The simplified malaria case definition agreed by WHO and partners for use in emergencies is summarized in Box 1.3. More detailed case definitions and classification for surveillance purposes are given in Chapter 3.

In all complex emergencies it is important to use a standardized case definition for malaria, in combination with a suitable rapid triage and screening process to identify those cases requiring immediate diagnosis and treatment. Basic confirmatory diagnostic capacity for malaria (using RDTs or microscopy) should be established as early as possible.

Box 1.3 **Simplified malaria case definition for use in emergencies**

Uncomplicated malaria
Person with fever or history of fever within the last 48 hours (with or without other symptoms such as nausea, vomiting and diarrhoea, headache, back pain, chills, myalgia), *where other obvious causes of fever have been excluded.*[1]

Severe malaria
Person with fever and symptoms as for uncomplicated malaria but with associated signs such as disorientation, loss of consciousness, convulsions, severe anaemia, jaundice, haemoglobinuria, spontaneous bleeding, pulmonary oedema, shock.

To confirm case
Demonstration of malaria parasites in blood films by examining thick or thin smears or by rapid diagnostic test for *P. falciparum*.

---

[1] In a high malaria risk area or season, all children under 5 years of age with fever (or history of fever) should be classified as having malaria (sometimes in addition to another febrile illness); presumptive treatment for malaria based on the clinical diagnosis is justified in this group given the high rate of malaria risk and the possibility that another illness might cause the malaria infection to progress.

In a low malaria risk area or season, children with fever (or history of fever) are classified as having malaria and given an antimalarial only if they have no runny nose (a sign of ARI), no measles and no other obvious cause of fever (pneumonia, sore throat, etc.). Parasitological confirmation in these children is recommended.

Malaria in complex emergencies

More than 80% of current complex emergencies are in malaria-endemic areas. A survey in eastern DRC showed that, during a period when violent deaths increased 5.5-fold, malaria-specific mortality increased 3.5-fold, including adult deaths (IRC, 2000). If this pattern is typical of the impact of sustained conflict, the number of deaths due to malaria in countries similarly affected by complex emergencies, such as Angola, Burundi, Guinea, Liberia, Sierra Leone, Somalia and Sudan, may be far higher than previously believed.

Populations at risk

In addition to the population groups generally at risk as identified above, others may be at increased risk of developing severe malaria during complex emergencies. The following factors all contribute to the increased malaria burden in affected populations:

— collapse of health services;
— ongoing conflict limiting access to effective treatment;
— resistance of the malaria parasites to commonly available drugs;
— lack of immunity to malaria; a population that has been displaced from a non-malarious area or an area of low transmission to (or through) an area of high transmission will have little immunity to the disease;
— weakened immunity because of multiple infections and malnutrition;
— exposure due to poor or absent housing;
— environmental deterioration resulting in increased vector breeding;
— population and parasite movement;
— poor knowledge among health agencies.

Some groups are particularly vulnerable, especially in the acute phase of a complex emergency, because they are given less priority in the distribution of limited resources, are marginalized socially or politically, or have greater difficulty in accessing treatment and care. Depending on the situation, these may include minority ethnic groups, older people, people with disabilities, and infants and children who are already weak or sick. Groups that are isolated from the main focus of humanitarian assistance are also vulnerable. For example, several hundred thousand refugees from Burundi and Rwanda fled from refugee camps around Goma, Bukavu and Uvira into the central forests of eastern DRC in 1997, because of fear of retribution. Several months passed before international assistance arrived. By this time, many children had died, and the prevalence of malaria and malnutrition was high. Tackling these issues of access can be extremely challenging.

Effective emergency response

The five principles of an effective emergency response, which apply both overall and to specific interventions such as malaria control, are:

- *Coordination* – among different partners to maximize overall capacity, promote linkages and complementary activities, and avoid duplication of effort. One emergency partner will normally take responsibility for coordination. This may be the ministry of health (in principle the first choice from the viewpoint of sustainability), the United Nations or a nongovernmental organization (NGO) and may change according to the situation and the stage of the emergency.
- *Accurate and timely assessment* – of the emergency situation and the needs of those affected (see Chapter 2).
- *Planning* – for the emergency response, based upon the results of assessment (see Chapter 2).
- *Implementation* – of the emergency response and specific interventions (see Chapters 3–7).
- *Monitoring and evaluation* – of the effectiveness of interventions by each emergency partner to ensure that programme activities are regularly reviewed and modified to maximize impact. Evaluation can be conducted by the agency implementing the interventions or, to increase objectivity, by an external organization.

Coordination among different partners

In emergencies, especially in conflict situations, international donors often terminate bilateral assistance to governments and focus on the delivery of humanitarian aid through international organizations, including United Nations agencies and international NGOs. These organizations are the key partners in emergency situations.

Operational partnerships between a range of organizations are essential in complex emergencies. It is critical to work with national and local government agencies, emergency organizations and personnel, wherever possible, when planning and implementing an emergency response. Existing health facilities and national staff can play an important role in emergency response and, with international support, are often best placed to deliver emergency health care.

Local NGOs and community groups are also important partners in the emergency response, usually after the acute phase, although they sometimes play a significant role early on. For example, AMIKIVU, a local NGO based in Goma, eastern DRC, has good diagnostic laboratory capacity. Working together with international partners, AMIKIVU diagnosed the first cholera cases in Rwandan refugees who fled to Goma in July 1994, and has continued to play an important support role in the overall emergency response since that time.

Local faith-based organizations also play a vital role in health care delivery in many countries. In DRC, for example, more than 80% of the country's health infrastructure is managed by Catholic and Protestant organizations.

Refugees, displaced people and war-affected resident populations often suffer from exhaustion, malnutrition and illness in the initial phase of an emergency. However, they have important skills, influence and cultural understanding, which may be lacking among the international humanitarian community, and it is important to identify the capacity that exists within affected populations as soon as possible and to work together with these populations.

Priorities and constraints

The priority in the acute phase of complex emergencies with high mortality rates is to establish effective life-saving interventions within the first few days. Interventions should be based on the best available evidence – both from existing information and from rapid assessment of the situation. The information gathered during assessment is essential, not only to plan appropriate interventions but also to lobby donor organizations for adequate funds. Emergency responses need to be tailored to the urgency of the situation, and unsustainable approaches are justified in the short-term until mortality rates are brought under control. Once the situation is stable, more sustainable approaches should be introduced, as the chronic phase of an emergency may go on for years.

It is important to remember that the ideal is not always possible in complex emergencies, especially in the acute phase; often there are significant constraints to delivering even basic interventions (see Box 1.4). These constraints affect what can be done, and organizations may have to make compromises in the way they manage patients, particularly inpatients. Within these constraints, however, every effort should be made to implement best practice. Poor quality interventions are never acceptable – they prolong suffering and result in unacceptable loss of life.

The international community may have to support rapid responses by providing expatriate staff and augmenting existing health infrastructure with temporary parallel facilities – such as mobile clinics and therapeutic

Box 1.4 **Constraints in complex emergencies**

The most common constraints encountered in complex emergencies are:

Health infrastructure
Local health facilities in complex emergencies are often in poor condition, as affected areas have frequently experienced many years of social and economic decline before the onset of conflict or political strife. Infrastructure may be destroyed during the emergency. Modern intensive care facilities and equipment, and even relatively basic inpatient equipment and supplies such as X-ray and oxygen, are rarely available or, if available, cannot be maintained in emergency conditions.

Capacity, human resources
During the acute phase of many complex emergencies, national capacity may be weakened and civil structures, including health and other services, are often unable to cope with the scale of response required. Shortages of skilled staff are the norm. Skilled national professionals, who have the means to leave, are often the first to be lost in conflict situations, further weakening national capacity. There is also a lack of the specific technical skills required to ensure health care delivery in difficult and challenging situations. Capacity may remain weak for many years.

Logistics
Supply, storage and distribution problems are exacerbated by poor road infrastructure, looting of stores, and breakdown of procurement systems and supply management.

Security
Poor security complicates logistics and service provision, restricts the access of vulnerable populations to health care, and places emergency teams under great stress, resulting in high staff turnover.

Funding
Delayed funding decisions, insufficient funding, and rapid decline in funding availability are key problems. Resources for training field teams in malaria control methods may also be severely limited.

Coordination
Lack of transparency, complementarity and information sharing among partners can hinder effective response.

feeding centres – to deal with additional and specific medical or operational management problems. Initial assessment should therefore include review of the capacity of existing health facilities in order to determine the staffing, and financial and material support required for an effective response.

Delivering effective malaria control responses

Effective malaria control in complex emergencies requires flexibility and innovation to maximize the impact of available resources. Large-scale funding made available in emergencies that have received wide media coverage may not be sustained beyond 6–12 months, and approaches used in the acute phase may not be feasible in the longer term. Programme design and strategies will need to be adapted through regular monitoring and review, in response to the changing situation.

Once mortality and morbidity rates are under control and have returned to pre-emergency levels, less intensive support may be required. Planning programme changes should be achieved through a careful process of reassessment and evaluation. If funding reductions are not appropriate, agencies will need to lobby donors with clear, evidence-based information to ensure effective health care for all those affected.

Reference

IRC (2000). *Mortality in eastern DRC: results from five mortality surveys by the International Rescue Committee*. Bukavu, International Rescue Committee.

Finding out more

An effective emergency response requires significant technical and operational skills. A list of resources and contact details is given in Annex I. Technical assistance and field support from RBM can also be obtained through:

Malaria in Emergencies Network
World Health Organization
1211 Geneva 27
Switzerland
Fax: +41 22 791 4824
E-mail: rbmemergencies@who.int

CHAPTER 2

Initial assessment and planning

This chapter:

■ outlines what information is essential and desirable for analysing the malaria burden and risk in emergency situations and planning and implementing an effective response

■ explains what to do if this information is not available, including how to conduct a rapid clinic-based fever survey and a rapid community cross-sectional prevalence survey

■ provides practical guidelines for selecting sites for displaced populations and managing drug supplies.

Understanding malaria

In an emergency situation, basic information about local malaria parasites, vectors, endemicity and transmission is desirable for the planning and implementation of appropriate and effective control measures. Country malaria profiles and communicable disease "toolkits" for many of the countries affected by emergencies can be found on the WHO/RBM web site (http://www.who.int/malaria/epidemicsandemergencies.html). Information on broader health issues is available in the country profiles generated and updated by WHO's Health Action in Crises department (www.who.int/hac). Country (malaria) profiles need to be regularly updated, especially from data generated by those working in the field.

In any malaria-endemic area, the following questions should be considered:

- Is it an area of high or low malaria transmission?
- Is there malaria transmission all year round or seasonal transmission?
- Are there malaria epidemics at particular times?

Assessment

In a complex emergency, a general assessment is essential to:

— identify current health priorities and potential health threats;

14

— assess the capacity and resources available to respond to the situation;

— collect baseline information for monitoring and evaluation of the effectiveness of planned interventions.

More specifically, it is important to determine the extent to which malaria is, or is likely to become, a major problem. Important questions to consider include:

- Is malaria a major health problem in the affected populations?
- Is the area prone to malaria outbreaks?
- Is there local transmission?
- Is malaria a major problem in the area from which the population has been displaced?
- Who is most at risk of malaria infection, illness and death?

Initial assessment of the situation should take less than a week, although this will depend on security, transport and communication. The information collected should be shared with other international and national emergency partners, so that it can contribute to the overall assessment both of the health situation and of wider humanitarian needs.

When conducting community malaria surveys or assessments at health facilities, it is essential to document both the presence of parasites (by RDT or microscopy) and clinical symptoms ("actual or reported fever" as a minimum). These data will provide useful information on both the proportion of symptomatic and asymptomatic malaria cases, and the proportion of febrile individuals without malaria.

Guiding principles for assessment, planning and selection of malaria control activities are summarized in Box 2.1

Box 2.1 **Guiding principles for assessment, planning and selection of malaria control activities**

- ■ Maximize the use of existing information at international, national, district and community levels.
- ■ Carry out rapid surveys if existing information is inadequate or inaccessible.
- ■ As far as possible, match malaria control interventions to current effective national policies, if known.
- ■ Use available local expertise to assist with the selection of malaria control options.
- ■ Involve affected populations in decision-making and action.

Obtaining information

Locally available data relevant to the emergency situation may be limited or outdated, particularly where government structures and services have been severely disrupted. If this is the case, it may be necessary to carry out rapid surveys, such as clinic-based fever surveys or cross-sectional prevalence surveys (details are given later in this chapter), to assess the situation and the relative importance of malaria. Carrying out malaria surveys at the same time as other rapid surveys, for example of nutritional status or vaccination coverage, can save time and money. In most emergency situations, there is uncertainty about:

— the actual malaria burden, due both to lack of mortality and morbidity data from the health services and to the absence of information about disease trends;
— the proportion of malaria cases (suspected and confirmed) that present for treatment at health facilities;
— the immune status of the refugee or displaced population, since there may be differences in malaria transmission in the areas that people have travelled through or settled in.

Information that is essential for early planning

When information is to be collected for planning, it is important to consider what information is critical and how it will be used to develop interventions. Information about the overall emergency situation, the population affected by the emergency, the malaria situation in the resettlement area and local capacity to respond is essential.

Emergency situation

Background information about the emergency situation and how it is likely to affect security and population movements is essential for planning interventions.

Affected population

Essential information about the affected population includes:

— estimated total population and breakdown by age and sex, and ongoing population movement (see Chapter 3);
— estimated mortality per 10 000 per day (see Chapter 3);
— immune status, population at risk for malaria, and emergency factors increasing vulnerability to malaria.

As discussed in Chapter 1, the level of immunity in a population depends on malaria endemicity (see Figure 2.1). Where people have been displaced, it is essential to find out where they have come from and whether or not they have travelled through malaria-endemic areas to reach the resettlement area. Groups within the displaced population may have different places of origin: some may have come from highly endemic areas, others from areas with little or no malaria transmission. Different groups may also have travelled along different routes and may or may not have been exposed to malaria during their journeys.

Figure 2.1 **Incidence of acute malaria infections (percentage by age) at different endemic levels in stable indigenous populations**

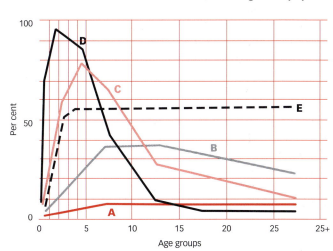

A Low endemicity. A person may attain adolescence before infection is acquired and may escape altogether.
B Moderate endemicity. Maximum incidence occurs in childhood and adolescence, but still not unusual for individuals to reach adulthood before acquiring infection.
C High endemicity. By late infancy or early childhood practically all are infected. Little acute illness in adolescents and still less in adults.
D Hyperendemicity. Most individuals acquire infection in early infancy, but acute manifestations are less frequent in childhood and are unusual in adults.
E Unless caused by exotic parasites, epidemics can occur only in populations where malaria was either previously absent or persisted at low or moderate endemic levels. They are characterized by a high incidence in all age groups (Boyd, 1949).

Malaria situation in the resettlement area
Morbidity caused by malaria

In order to prioritize interventions and monitor their effectiveness, it is essential to discover how much morbidity, including severe anaemia, in the target population is due to malaria, and which population and age groups are most affected. The age groups most affected will indicate pre-existing population immunity levels – and thus endemicity in the areas from which the population originated – but may also indicate age groups at particular risk of transmission, for example adult men who stay overnight in forested areas in some Asian countries where transmission is intense.

This information can be obtained from provincial, national, district and local levels by the following means:

- A review of past and present medical records – suspected and confirmed malaria morbidity data and, if available, severe anaemia data (haemoglobin <6 g/dl), disease trends and surveillance data) – from the affected locations.
- A rapid fever survey at a health facility or mobile clinic, preferably one that sees patients from all affected groups (i.e. host, refugee and internally displaced). Such a survey will indicate the actual proportion of confirmed malaria cases among people who perceive themselves to be sick with a febrile disease.

Mortality caused by malaria

Specific mortality data are usually unavailable or, for various reasons, are inaccurate. Data on case-fatality rate (CFR) could be obtained in referral hospitals or facilities that admit patients with severe disease, bearing in mind that such data represent only a fraction of the real mortality at community level and tend to reflect the quality of case management in health care facilities. Surveys using questionnaires can be used in camps or communities to provide more accurate specific estimates of mortality and burden of disease.

Malaria endemicity and transmission

Information about the local level of malaria endemicity and patterns of malaria transmission (see Chapter 1) should be obtained from data available either within the country or from elsewhere (e.g. WHO). It is also important to know about geographical and climatic factors that affect endemicity and transmission, such as seasonal variations in rainfall and temperature.

Malaria outbreaks and malaria control efforts

It is essential to find out whether there are any known risk factors for malaria outbreaks – for example, a large influx of non-immune people into an area of high transmission, rainfall after an unusual period of drought, recent environmental changes that have increased suitable breeding sites – and whether the area has experienced earlier outbreaks. If there have been earlier outbreaks, it is important to find out whether the numbers of people affected and the causes of the outbreak were documented, and to be aware of past and present malaria control efforts in the area, so that these efforts can be built on and lessons learned from past experiences.

Malaria parasite species

The malaria parasite species present in the area and the relative importance of each must be determined: this information will affect the choice of control measures and possibly the choice of treatment (see Chapter 1). Information on malaria species could be obtained from laboratory records or – for greater accuracy – from a cross-sectional parasitological survey.

Local vectors, vector behaviour, susceptibility to main insecticides and suitable breeding sites

The following questions should be considered:

- Are there malaria vectors present?
- What vector species are they, where do they like to breed, and when and where do they feed?
- Do they prefer humans or animals?
- What are the vector resting patterns?
- Where do people come into contact with the vector and under what conditions?

Information about local vectors, their biting and resting habits, and their susceptibility to insecticides is critical (see Chapter 1 and refer to Tables 6.6–6.9). The local vector species affect transmission patterns and consequently the choice of cost-effective vector control options. It may be useful to find out about the location of major breeding sites, for example, areas that are badly drained, marshy, low-lying and prone to flooding, and that are close to where people live. This information is particularly useful at the early stage, to avoid siting camps in high-risk areas, and later for selecting potential additional prevention measures.

Information on local vectors is often difficult to obtain but could be gathered from:

— the ministry of health and the national malaria control programme, if accessible;
— records from previous entomological surveys (see reports or "grey" literature maintained in international institutions such as WHO);
— published literature such as the information on malaria vectors compiled by Mouchet et al. (2002).

Capacity to respond

The capacity to respond to the emergency will often depend on international and national partners. It is important to assess the presence and activities of other agencies and mechanisms and scope for co-ordination and joint planning. You also need to assess the capacity of health services and to review national policy and regulations regarding drugs and insecticides.

Health infrastructure and personnel

The condition of public and private health facilities and other infrastructure should be assessed, as should the availability of personnel, particularly those who have worked in malaria control (see the checklist in Table 2.1). This assessment should include the type of health facilities, the number of

Table 2.1 **Health system condition**

System	Present (Y/N)	Fee system (Y/N)	Observations
1. Clinical diagnosis			
2. IMCI[a] strategy in use in country			
3. Laboratory diagnosis			
4. Treatment of uncomplicated malaria			
5. Referral system and facilities			
6. Transport facilities			
7. Management of severe malaria			
8. Previous use of insecticide-treated materials among refugees and host population			
9. Other vector control			
10. Monitoring and surveillance			

[a] Integrated Management of Childhood Illness.

health workers and their level of training, referral services, availability of diagnostic facilities, drugs and equipment (including blood transfusion facilities), the effectiveness of communication between different levels of the system, and whether or not a surveillance system exists.

Accessibility and use of health services

It is important to find out about the host population's access to, and use of, existing health care services, and the extent to which these services could be strengthened to serve the displaced or refugee population. Factors that are likely to reduce access and treatment-seeking behaviour significantly in emergencies include poor security, culturally inappropriate services, preferences for alternative sources of health care, and charging partially or fully (cost recovery) for consultation, diagnosis and treatment. It should be kept in mind that, in most refugee camps supported by humanitarian agencies, access to health care is usually free of charge.

Drugs and insecticides

National policies and regulations govern the use of drugs and insecticides in all countries, so it is important to find out:

— what antimalarial drugs (see Chapter 5) are currently recommended by the ministry of health for treatment of uncomplicated malaria and for management of severe malaria, as well as what other drugs are used locally;
— whether potential emergency drug options are registered or whether this will need to be negotiated and introduced;
— what insecticides (see Chapter 6) are recommended and used;
— what evidence is available for the efficacy of drugs and insecticides being used under national protocols.

Information to be collected after initial assessment

After the initial emergency assessment, sufficient basic information should be available to allow immediate priority interventions to be started. However, to develop the emergency response and improve the impact of control activities, additional information should be collected to inform planning.

Health policy, planning and services

Information on the treatment-seeking behaviour of the population and on health care provision by traditional healers and private practitioners is critical in order to ensure that planned interventions will actually deliver effective treatment to those in need. Planning should include working with private treatment providers if these are commonly used by the population that will be served.

Information is needed on current health sector reforms and financial mechanisms, health service logistics, and responsibilities for planning and implementation at national, regional, provincial and district levels.

Malaria control programme

It is important to find out about the national malaria control programme – goals, objectives, targets and action plans; structure, management and staff; guidelines, including those on dealing with malaria in emergencies and epidemics; and current control efforts.

Other priority programmes and activities

Information should be gathered on the national essential drugs list; drug stocks, supply and distribution systems; environmental health activities (e.g. vector control, insecticide stocks and supply lines); mother and child health initiatives, such as Making Pregnancy Safer, and Integrated Management of Childhood Illness (IMCI); and information management systems.

Displaced or refugee and host populations

Other information that is essential is related to: population movement, settlement patterns and occupations; knowledge, attitudes and beliefs among different ethnic groups about malaria and its causes, prevention and treatment; and current level of usage of protective measures such as insecticide-treated materials, types of shelter and, where possible, family sleeping arrangements.

Important considerations in complex emergencies

In addition to factors that increase the vulnerability of the affected populations to malaria, such as malnutrition, anaemia, co-infections, and limited housing facilities, it is also important to investigate the following situations, which can result in high rates of malaria mortality and morbidity:

— movement from areas of high transmission to areas of low or no malaria transmission
— movement from areas of low or no transmission to areas of high malaria transmission
— movement to areas with different malaria species.

Movement from areas of high transmission to areas of low or no malaria transmission

If the refugee or displaced population has moved from or through an area of high malaria transmission to an area of low or no malaria transmission, there may be explosive outbreaks in the non-immune host population, depending on the malaria receptivity status (possibility of transmission) of the region (see Box 2.2). In this situation, all patients with fever should be checked for malaria using either microscopic examination or RDTs, otherwise malaria cases will be missed and misdiagnosed.

Careful analysis is essential: the risk to the host population is sometimes overestimated because of the large number of malaria episodes in the arriving population. It is equally important not to discount the risk to the host population given its lack of immunity. The arriving population may have a higher incidence of disease episodes than they had been used to at home, simply as a result of the stress of displacement.

Box 2.2 **High malaria prevalence in an area of low transmission**

> Over two months in 1994, some 500 000 refugees from Rwanda settled in Ngara camp in the United Republic of Tanzania. Although the camp was in an area of low malaria transmission, the prevalence of malaria among refugees was very high and many people died from the disease. This was because the refugees had passed through an endemic region of Rwanda on their way to Ngara and became sick only once they had arrived at the camp. The proportion of febrile patients with falciparum parasites reached a peak prevalence of 35% after the first 4 weeks of resettlement and subsequently declined, stabilizing at 11%.

Over time, the proportion of the refugee or displaced population that is infected – and related malaria mortality and morbidity – will decline unless the introduction of infected anopheline mosquitoes into the area leads to an outbreak. However, it is important to remember that malaria parasites can stay in the blood for a considerable time. Their persistence depends on the species: *P. falciparum* parasites usually remain in the blood for less than one year, while *P. malariae* and *P. vivax* may persist for years.

If refugees or displaced people return to their area of origin after a period of more than a year, it should be assumed that they have lost most of their semi-immune status. Children born in the camp will be especially at risk once they return "home".

Movement from areas of low or no transmission to areas of high malaria transmission

If the refugee or displaced population has moved from an area of low or no malaria transmission to an area of high malaria transmission, all age groups are at risk. Mortality rates may be high (see Box 2.3). In this context, and after the exclusion of other prevalent infectious diseases, all fever cases should be considered as potentially due to malaria and should, wherever possible, be confirmed by laboratory diagnosis and then treated (see Chapter 5).

Movement to areas with different malaria species

Populations may be immune to species of malaria parasite that are prevalent in their areas of origin, but they will be at increased risk if they move to an area where a different species, to which they have little or no immunity, predominates.

Epidemiological investigation methods

Epidemiological investigation is required to determine whether malaria is, or may become, a significant problem and to monitor trends. This is particularly important when the local malaria situation is not clearly defined (see Figure 2.2). For example, a high proportion of fever cases and associated deaths during the acute phase of an emergency suggests that malaria may be an important problem. If the malaria burden is very high in all age groups, this may either indicate that the refugee or displaced or host populations have developed little or no immunity, or signal the beginning of an outbreak (see Chapter 4).

> *Note:* There is no specific epidemiological threshold for a malaria outbreak; thresholds must be adjusted to each epidemiological situation. However, the early stage of an outbreak is usually characterized by a high and rapidly increasing number of people who are sick with fever due to malaria, and a high proportion (usually >50%) of febrile patients who are infected with malaria parasites.

Rapid surveys

Rapid surveys are essential to:

— estimate the proportion of the population, both symptomatic and asymptomatic, infected with *P. falciparum* and other species;
— identify population groups most at risk;
— determine priorities for action, including the most appropriate case management and vector control measures.

24

Box 2.3 **High malaria mortality in non-immune populations moving
to high-transmission areas**

In Rwanda in 1993, many people were forced to move from highland areas
in the north of the country, where there is no malaria transmission, to the
lowlands in the centre of the country, where malaria transmission is high.
During the same year, refugees from highland areas of Burundi started to
move to Kigoma in the United Republic of Tanzania, where malaria is highly
endemic. In both situations, mortality rates were high in the incoming non-
immune population.

Figure 2.2 **Assessing the risk of malaria**

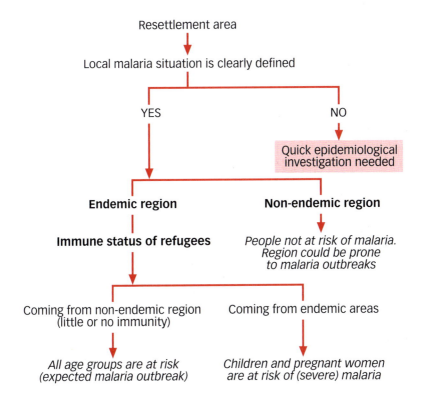

They include:

— clinic-based fever survey at a health facility or mobile clinic;
— cross-sectional prevalence survey across the affected population(s).

Rapid surveys assess basic clinical signs and parasite presence using microscopy or RDTs (see Box 2.4). They can be carried out at health centre level by confirmatory testing of symptomatic patients (patients with febrile illness or a history of fever), to determine the proportion of febrile cases due to malaria. In acute emergencies, when caseloads are unusually high, clinic-based surveys can provide a very useful initial indication of the relative importance of malaria as a cause of morbidity at facility level. However, it is not enough just to survey outpatients with fever, because data from health facilities provide information only about people who seek treatment at those facilities. In well set up refugee camps where health care is provided free of charge, it is possible that everybody can access health care (usually 5–10 times more than in "normal" conditions); in less well organized situa-

---

Box 2.4 **Definitions**

Positive RDT rate
The proportion of RDTs positive for *P. falciparum* malaria. Depending on the test used (for example with the HRP-II test), RDT results tend to stay positive for 1–2 weeks after completion of treatment.

Parasite rate or slide positivity rate (SPR) or positive RDT rate in patients presenting with febrile disease or suspected malaria
The proportion of patients presenting with fever or history of fever in the past 48 hours who have malaria parasites in their blood. For the purposes of a rapid prevalence survey, malaria disease is defined as fever (axillary temperature ≥37.5 °C) or history of fever in the past 48 hours *plus* the presence of malaria parasites.

Parasite rate or SPR or positive RDT rate in the population
The proportion of blood films or RDTs showing parasites in a given resident population (preferably in the age group 2–9 years).

Spleen rate
The proportion of enlarged spleens (splenomegaly) in a given population (preferably in the age group 2–9 years). In a child with a distended abdomen from intestinal parasitosis, the umbilicus cannot be used as a guide for spleen measurement. It is important to remember that there may be other causes of splenomegaly in the area (e.g. visceral leishmaniasis or schistosomiasis). It should be noted that increased access to antimalarial drugs has an impact on the spleen rate in the investigated population.

tions, only a minority of the people who are actually sick may attend facilities. The data will not be representative of the overall population nor will they provide any indication of what proportion of the overall population has malaria infection; cross-sectional prevalence surveys in the community are necessary. Depending on the population of interest, the community may be the displaced or refugee population and/or the host population. It may be necessary to repeat the community survey in different sites if there are reasons to suspect localized variations in malaria epidemiology and there is limited contact between the different populations.

Rapid clinic-based fever survey at a health facility

The purpose of a clinic survey is to find out the prevalence of parasitaemia among symptomatic patients attending the clinic, i.e. the proportion of febrile patients with malaria parasites.

Conducting the survey

- Choose microscopy or RDTs. In an environment where there are usually no skilled microscopists, RDTs give reliable and quick results – always bearing in mind that some manufactured tests may be of poor quality, which will affect the sensitivity and specificity of the malaria diagnosis. Microscopy through proper staining procedures and under supervision by skilled microscopists remains the gold standard for malaria diagnosis in addition to the fact that blood smears remain intact for months and can be checked (quality control – assurance) by supervisors outside the population area. Ensure that assessment team staff are adequately trained and skilled to use the chosen method.
- Ensure that there are sufficient staff.
- Select a health facility or mobile clinic(s) with high patient attendance. Test all patients presenting with a febrile illness, using microscopy or RDTs, up to at least 100 patients. If possible do this in one day.
- Record the total number of outpatients seen at the clinic while the survey is being done.
- Record the age, sex and place of origin of all patients and the pregnancy status of female patients.
- Use the definition of malaria-positive described in Box 2.4 (parasite rate or SPR or positive RDT rate in patients presenting with febrile disease or suspected malaria).
- In the first few weeks of the acute phase, repeat the survey every week, and then at least every month to monitor trends.

Analysis and use of results
- Record the total number of patients at the clinic, total number of fever cases, proportion of fever cases among all outpatients, and proportion of confirmed malaria cases among fever cases investigated.
- Present the results graphically by week and age group.

In the host population
- If parasites are found in fewer than 10% of fever cases, this is an indication of low transmission (children and adults usually at risk of disease).
- If parasites are found in more than 50% of fever cases in children aged under 10 years and less than 50% of adult fever cases, this is an indication of high transmission (children most at risk).
- If parasites are found in more than 50% of fever cases in children aged over 10 years and adults, this is an indication of the possible onset of an outbreak.

In the refugee population
Analysis in the refugee population is more complex, since the same results may reflect different scenarios or situations (as listed below), especially in the first few weeks of settlement. A high proportion of fever cases positive for malaria in refugees or displaced people may be an indication of:
- High local malaria transmission:
  — If the incoming population is non-immune, high morbidity and mortality rates will be recorded in all age groups.
  — If the incoming population is semi-immune, children and pregnant women are most at risk, showing high morbidity and mortality rates.
- High malaria endemicity in the area of origin, regardless of the level of transmission in the resettlement area:
  — If there is low transmission in the resettlement area, over time either local transmission may start on an epidemic scale if receptivity is high or fewer and fewer people will become sick until there is a low proportion of malaria disease in health care facilities.
- High malaria endemicity in areas they travelled through regardless of the level of transmission in the resettlement area:
  — As above.
- The beginning of a malaria outbreak if the refugees or displaced population have come from a low to a high transmission area.

Rapid cross-sectional fever and parasitological prevalence survey across the affected population

Guiding principles

- Highly precise survey results are usually not needed during acute emergencies. The need is rather for acceptable precision in determining the level of malaria endemicity, particularly to distinguish between medium/high endemicity (more than 10% of people in the general population are infected) and low endemicity (well under 10% of people are infected), since the interventions to be planned are quite different.

- More precise survey data may be needed for operational research and for evaluating the impact of interventions over time and space.

The purpose of a community cross-sectional prevalence survey is to:

— provide pre-intervention baseline data;
— ascertain the prevalence of symptomatic and asymptomatic malaria (with confirmed parasitaemia) across all age groups;
— identify groups at risk and target interventions;
— gather information on the treatment-seeking behaviour of the population, for example, whether they received treatment in the previous 7 days, what treatment they received and where they received it.

In general, it can take 3–6 days to carry out a rapid cross-sectional malaria prevalence survey and it should be planned accordingly. It is useful to collect baseline information about haemoglobin levels (for example, using the Haemoglobin Colour Scale) where possible, because malaria is often an important cause of severe anaemia (Hb <6 g/dl) in endemic areas.

Conducting the survey

- *Choose a diagnostic tool.* Unless there is a team of good microscopists, RDTs (pre-qualified, once available, or with evidence of good manufacturing practice; www.wpro.who.int/rdt) are the most appropriate tools for testing the blood for malaria parasites where rapid results are needed. Several RDTs are available, but the stability of all of them is affected by conditions of high humidity and temperature (>30 °C). Some test only for *P. falciparum* while others will test for more than one species but are usually more expensive and less stable than tests for *P. falciparum* alone. Cassettes and cards are simpler to use than dipsticks, but all need basic training and regular supervision. Microscopy can be used if sufficient time, resources and trained staff are available and if there is a need to determine the prevalence of other species and to establish and maintain quality control procedures.

- *Define the study population.* If there are differences in malaria epidemiology, it will be necessary to define a study population within each type of ecological area or to take separate samples of the same size from each area.

- *Determine the sample size.* The required sample size depends on the expected prevalence of malaria illness and parasitaemia, on how precise the results need to be (i.e. how "wide" the 95% confidence interval can be allowed to be), on the sampling method (the "design effect") and, to a lesser extent, on the size of the population. For valid comparisons, a smaller sample is sufficient when the spleen or parasite rate is high in the investigated areas. For statistical validity of results, however, a large sample is required; see example in Table 2.2. The StatCalc program on EpiInfo, which can be downloaded free from http://www.cdc.gov/epiinfo, can be used to help in the calculation of sample size.

For example:

The prevalence is assumed to be 50%; 45% is used as the "lowest acceptable result"; the population is 25 000; the chosen confidence interval is 95%. The desirable sample size using EpiInfo would be 378. With an assumed design effect of 2 (depending on the sampling method), the required sample size is 2 x 378 = 756.

Table 2.2 **Confidence interval at 95% probability level for a standardized sample of 100 and 500, using random sampling**

Prevalence	60	50	40	10	5
95% confidence interval, with a sample size at random of 100	50–70	40–60	30–50	5–18	2–11
95% confidence interval, with a sample size at random of 500	56–64	46–54	36–44	8–13	3–7

For example:

If in a sample of 100 children parasites are found in 50, the parasite rate in the total population of children of the same age group lies between 40% and 60%, and this may be assumed with a 95% probability. With the same result in a sample of 500 children, the 95% confidence interval would be 46–54% (Bruce-Chwatt, 1985).

Note: These figures are for random sampling, *not* for cluster sampling. Random sampling selects sample units such that each possible unit has a fixed and determinate probability of selection (Last, 2001). Thus, each person has an equal chance of being selected out of the total study population. Random sampling should not be confused with haphazard assignment. Random sampling follows a predetermined plan that is usually devised with the aid of a table of random numbers.

- *Confidence interval.* A 95% confidence interval is the standard bench-mark used when analysing survey data. It means that there is a less than 5% chance that the true values will fall outside the interval. The larger the sample size, the more accurate is the measured prevalence rate expected to be, and the narrower the 95% confidence interval. Survey reports should preferably provide a 95% confidence interval in the results. Confidence intervals can become fairly wide when data need to be broken down by age – which is probably adequate for purposes of planning malaria control programmes. However, to demonstrate a statistically significant change in prevalence associated with a particular intervention, the size of the effect would need to be very large to be detected. If the results from the study are to show that an intervention has been effective, a larger sample size may be needed. This is particularly important for children under 5 years of age, because it is often this group that should be targeted by interventions and the desired changes associated with these interventions need to be measured.

- *Choose a sampling method.* There are many sampling methods. For malaria, everyone in the household is usually surveyed. Each household must have an equal chance of being selected. Methods of selecting households include random sampling, systematic sampling, and random cluster sampling. However, in the acute phase of emergencies, households may not be stable or well defined, and the most appropriate method in the first few weeks of this phase may be random sampling.

- *Recruit and train survey team, selecting one person as team leader.* The team should include:
  — 1 person to explain the procedure and obtain informed consent from the household. Ideally this person should be a community member.
  — 1 person to register the participants, record the axillary temperature, the RDT result and information on treatment-seeking behaviour.
  — 1 person to take the axillary temperature and perform the RDT or make a malaria smear on a slide.
  — 1 person to measure spleen size (if this is to be done) or, more feasible in emergencies, to check for the presence of enlarged spleen.
  — 1 person to administer treatment (if this is given on the spot) and to provide advice about danger signs and follow-up.

- *Ensure adequate supplies.* The following are essential:
  — Rapid tests or microscope slides and associated consumables (e.g. lancets, rubber gloves, alcohol for swabbing skin, cotton wool, suitable disposal facilities for sharps and contaminated materials).

— Referral forms for the nearest suitable clinic.
— Administrative equipment, e.g. log book, consent forms (see an example in Annex II), record forms (see Annex III), pens, pencils and markers.
— Funds to pay for transport to the clinic if needed.

• *Repeat the survey.* It can be useful to repeat the survey during a different season and compare the results, if malaria transmission is seasonal. For example, in some areas prevalence is lower at the end of the dry season than at the end of the wet season. In areas where malaria transmission is intense all year round, repeating the survey several months after the start of the emergency response can provide a good indication of the impact of interventions. In areas with marked seasonal peaks it may be useful to repeat the survey after 12 months (i.e. at the same time of year) to measure any impact of interventions.

Analysis and use of results

• *Prevalence of malaria.* Calculate the proportion of people, out of the entire population, with fever or a history of fever who have a positive RDT (or slide) result. This will provide an estimate of the prevalence of malaria in the study population at that specific point in time. Analyse the data by sex and by age group. The number of pregnant women in the sample will probably be too low to be statistically significant.

• *Endemicity.* Calculate the proportion of people who have a positive RDT or slide result and the proportion who have splenomegaly (bearing in mind that widespread use of drugs may affect splenomegaly rate). Use the parasite rates – or spleen rates if microscopy or RDTs are not possible – to estimate the underlying endemicity of malaria (see Table 2.3).

Table 2.3 **Malaria endemicity according to spleen and parasite rates**

Malaria endemicity	Spleen rate (SR)		Parasite rate (PR)	
	Under 5 years	Over 5 years	Under 5 years	Over 5 years
Meso- and hyper-endemic (usually linked to high transmission)	Very high	Low or zero	High (>50%), but lower than spleen rate	Low
Hypoendemic (usually linked to low transmission)	Low (<10%)		≤10%, always higher than spleen rate	

In cross-sectional surveys, parasite and spleen rates are normally determined in children aged 2–9 years. In areas where malaria transmission is high, parasite and spleen rates are highest in children aged under 5 years and decline above that age. In areas where malaria transmission is low, parasite and spleen rates are low and are equally distributed over all age groups.

- *Representativeness of the sample.* Check the survey data to see whether there are many absentees, whether the sex and age of absentees are statistically different from the group sampled, and whether particular groups (e.g. children aged under 5 years) are underrepresented. Also review the sex and age groups of the sample to see whether the proportions are similar to those in the whole community (see Chapter 3, Table 3.1).

- Enter the data into a software program (e.g. EpiInfo) to help with analysis.

- Calculate to 95% confidence interval, if possible.

Important aspects of planning
Selecting resettlement sites
In the initial phase of complex emergencies, refugees and internally displaced people move quickly to the nearest safe place outside the conflict area. Subsequently, international organizations and the host government may resettle the refugee or displaced population in more permanent sites. Whether or not this happens depends on the local situation; for example, some host governments may be reluctant to encourage the establishment of long-term settlements.

If refugees and displaced populations are to be resettled, criteria for selecting a site include the availability of water and land, means of transport, access to fuel, security and, where relevant, distance from borders. However, areas that meet these criteria are usually already occupied by the resident population, so refugees and displaced populations are often resettled in less desirable sites.

If there is a choice, it may be necessary to consider more specific criteria that may affect the risk of malaria (see Box 2.5). When selecting a site:

- Assess the epidemiological characteristics of the area, if this information is available.

- Investigate potential vector breeding sites and make use of local expertise and knowledge of local vectors.

- Avoid sites close to major breeding places of local vectors. In Africa, such sites often include marshy areas and flat, low-lying land at risk of flooding. If possible, sloping, well-drained sites with tree cover, sheltered from strong winds, should be chosen. In south-east Asia, thick forest should be avoided.

Box 2.5 **Malaria and resettlement sites**

In 1994, around 1 million people fled from Rwanda to eastern DRC in a short period of time. Four refugee camps were established around the town of Goma. One of these camps was sited close to lowland marshes. Malaria prevalence in this camp was 30–40%, compared with 5–15% in the other three camps, resulting in high rates of mortality.

Selecting vector control activities

If malaria transmission is very high, rapid prescriptive standardized approaches, may be necessary, such as indoor residual spraying (IRS), or provision of blankets or other materials that have been treated with insecticide (see Chapter 6). However, costly activities such as IRS require a clear understanding of vector behaviour and the susceptibility of the vectors to insecticides.

Selecting effective first-line antimalarial treatment

Since early diagnosis and prompt effective treatment are the first priority in malaria control, it is essential to select and use a first-line antimalarial drug that is efficacious and safe, with limited contraindications and side-effects (see Chapter 5).

Managing supplies of antimalarial and other essential drugs

After antimalarials have been selected, important steps in establishing systems to manage drug supplies are the following:

- Establishment of a working group or interagency committee, involving local and international agencies and organizations, to manage the emergency.

- Establishment of a subcommittee of the working group to manage supplies of essential drugs, including antimalarials. It makes sense for the agency with the most experience and expertise in essential drug supply management to take the lead, with responsibility for receiving, storing and distributing drugs and monitoring drug supply. However, it is also important to respect the sovereignty of the host country and the affected population, regardless of the drug supply situation.

- Careful attention to drug quality and sources of supply. It is important to check product specifications, expiry dates, dosage form and strengths.

- Proper management of stocks. Drugs from different sources should be easily identifiable or kept separately. The system for stock management should be as simple as possible and within the scope of the host country. If the complex emergency is very severe or large scale, it may be necessary to computerize the stock management system.

- Development of a clear policy for free distribution of drugs, ensuring that all agencies and communities are aware of this policy.

- Ensuring that all staff who provide health care are trained in rational use of drugs, including recommended antimalarials; provision of training if necessary.

- Getting the advice of the relevant authorities if donated supplies or the only available supplies of drugs are not approved or included in national protocols. If there is no other option, staff should be trained in the rational use of these drugs as a temporary measure to save lives; approved treatment guidelines should be used as soon as this is possible.

- Ensuring that patients are followed up where possible. This requires adequate staff and a good patient registration system. Patient follow-up may not be feasible in the acute phase of an emergency where there are large caseloads, but should be possible once the displaced or refugee population is living in stable settlements and during the chronic phase. If possible, the opportunity should be taken to monitor patient drug use behaviour, for example adherence to treatment regimens.

- Early decision, with the host government, on whether or not the resident population will also have access to health care services delivered as part of humanitarian assistance. If so, estimates of the resident population must be included when drug supply requirements are calculated.

Summary

- Assess the existing capacity and data:
  — pre-departure data collection (24 hours)
  — general assessment in the field (less than 1 week).

- Find out what proportion of people presenting to the clinic with a febrile illness have malaria:
  — clinic-based fever survey (1 day).

- Find out how big the problem is and who is most affected:
  — rapid cross-sectional malaria prevalence survey (3–6 days).

- Define intervention on the basis of the results of the rapid surveys in health care facilities and through household surveys, taking into account as well other important risk factors (such as severe malnutrition) and operational information gathered through the first assessments.

References

Boyd MF, ed. (1949). *Malariology. A comprehensive survey of all aspects of this group of diseases from a global standpoint.* Philadelphia, Saunders.

Bruce-Chwatt LJ (1985). *Essential malariology*, 2nd ed. London, Heinemann Medical Books.

Last JM, ed. (2001). *A dictionary of epidemiology*, 4th ed. New York, Oxford University Press.

Mouchet J et al. (2004). *Biodiversité du paludisme dans le monde [Biodiversity of malaria worldwide].* Montrouge, France, John Libley Eurotext.

Finding out more

Most of the information you require for initial assessment can usually be obtained from:

— interviews with health authorities, government representatives, members of the affected community, health care personnel, donor and United Nations agency representatives, and health care agencies;

— review of reception and registration records;

— laboratory records;

— published literature;

— reports from WHO and international partners.

Sources of information to help with planning include WHO, United Nations Children's Fund (UNICEF), United Nations Development Programme (UNDP), Office of the United Nations High Commissioner for Refugees (UNHCR), health ministries and national malaria control programmes, research institutions, NGOs, international and national journals and publications and web sites (see Annex I).

CHAPTER 3

Surveillance

This chapter:
- outlines the information that is needed to plan and implement a surveillance system to monitor the ongoing malaria situation
- describes how to establish a surveillance system, including the data that should be collected, how to collect them and how to use them.

Malaria surveillance in complex emergencies

Surveillance is the continual and systematic collection, analysis and interpretation of health data essential to the planning, implementation and evaluation of health interventions. It is also a tool for measuring the health status of a population. In a complex emergency situation, surveillance is a priority and must be established quickly. It can, for example, help both to determine whether or not malaria is a significant health problem and to decide on operational priorities.

Malaria surveillance should be integrated into an overall system for surveillance of all the main causes of mortality, which is usually based on the network of health facilities in an area.

The purpose of malaria surveillance is to:

- *Monitor trends*, for example:
  Are malaria cases or malaria deaths increasing or decreasing?
  Is this due to new arrivals or the displacement of the population?

- *Provide early warning of an outbreak*, for example:
  Is malaria incidence increasing?

- *Monitor the effectiveness of malaria control interventions and, if necessary, redefine priorities*, for example:
  Do sick people have access to health care?
  How effective is detection and treatment of malaria cases?

If no surveillance system is in place or the existing system is inadequate, it is essential to establish a system – but this must be done in a coordinated way (see Box 3.1). Obstacles to establishing a surveillance system in a complex emergency situation may include:

— poor understanding at field level of what a surveillance system is and why it is needed, resulting in poor recording, reporting and use of information;
— poor motivation of health workers because of lack of feedback;
— lack of diagnostic tools to confirm clinical diagnosis, resulting in inaccurate and unreliable data;
— lack of representativeness of data collected because only a small percentage of the population use health services and security problems limit access for a proportion of the affected population;
— lack of coordination between agencies.

Box 3.1 **Surveillance problems in East Timor[1]**

Following a vote for independence from Indonesia in August 1999, most of the population of East Timor[1] was displaced, and health facilities and medical infrastructure were destroyed. There was no functioning government or ministry of health, records had been destroyed and there were no available data. All humanitarian and health agencies began to develop their own basic surveillance systems to collect baseline data about disease incidence, prevalence and mortality rates to enable them to plan health services. Coordination was poor, however, and information was not always shared. Eventually a standardized surveillance system was developed by WHO.

[1] Now Timor-Leste.

Collecting basic information

Before a surveillance system is implemented, certain basic information about the size and structure of the population is essential. It can also be useful to find out about recent mortality.

Population size

To be able to calculate health indicators, such as the mortality rate, the total size of the population must be known. This can be determined by:

— counting households and the average number of people per household
— mapping the site's surface area and measuring the average population density

— carrying out a census or reviewing records of camp registration, food distribution, etc; or

— using information from programme activities (e.g. vaccine coverage).

Counting households

The total size of a population is estimated by multiplying the number of households by the average number of people per household: this information can be obtained by exhaustive counting or systematic sampling.

Exhaustive counting of households

1. Count the total number of households in the area. This can be done on foot, from a vehicle or by aerial photography. Because it is exhaustive, this method is most appropriate for small sites covering limited areas.
2. Calculate the average number of persons per household by conducting a small survey of sample households selected at random. A minimum of 30 households should be selected.
3. Estimate the total population by multiplying the total number of households by the average number of persons per household.

Systematic sampling

1. This technique is particularly adapted to well-organized refugee camps. Using interval sampling and a departure number chosen at random, select a sample (and thus determine each household to be visited). This method assumes that households are arranged in such a way that interval sampling is possible and that their approximate number is known.

   For example:
   Estimated no. of household = 4000
   Convenient sample size chosen = 400
   Sample interval = 4000/400 = 10 (information on the number of person living in an household will be collected in every 10 habitats)

   If the randomly chosen departure point is 6 (i.e. the sixth household beginning at one extremity of the camp), the selected households are therefore number 6, then number 16 (6+10), then number 26 (16+10), etc.

2. Estimate the total population by multiplying:
   (total no. of households visited) x (average no. of persons per household) x sample interval.

Mapping

The total size of a population is estimated by multiplying the total surface area of a site (m^2) by the average population density per m^2: this information can be obtained by the quadrate method or the T-square method.

Quadrate method (see Figure 3.1)

1. Draw the camp boundary. This can be accomplished either by taking GPS points along the perimeter and drawing the map with software, or by hand with a compass and then on paper.
2. Select 30 systematically random locations within the site. This can also be accomplished by mapping software or by hand. In Figure 3.1, six such points are shown.
3. Mark off a 25 m x 25 m quadrate, or block, physically with a rope or using a telemeter at each point.
4. Count the population within each quadrate, and the number of persons and number of households for the 30 quadrates.
5. Calculate the average population per quadrate.
6. Estimate the site population by extrapolating the average population per quadrate to the entire site surface. Confidence intervals are then calculated around the estimate.

Figure 3.1 **Quadrate method for calculating population size**[a]

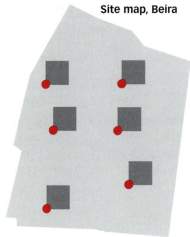

Site map, Beira

1. Draw site boundary
2. Select 30 starting points
3. Mark 30 (25 m x 25 m) blocks
4. Count population in each block
5. Calculate average population/block
6. Estimate the total site population

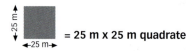

= 25 m x 25 m quadrate

[a] Source: MSF/Epicentre.

Further details for the quadrate method are provided in *Rapid health assessment of refugee or displaced populations* (MSF, 2005, in press).

T-square method[1]

The T-square method "involves sampling a number of random points, measuring the distance between each point and the nearest household or family unit, and then measuring the distance between that household and the next closest one, as a way of measuring population density".[2] It gives a more accurate evaluation of the population size, but is more complicated to perform than the quadrate method.

Census or registration

Census

A census of the displaced population is the ideal method, if it is feasible. It involves visiting homes and counting how many people live in each. If security allows, it is best done early in the morning or in the evening when refugees or displaced people are "at home". However, in an emergency situation, there may not be sufficient time or human resources to carry out a census.

> For example:
> Following the floods in Mozambique, a quick census was carried out by an agency in two temporary accommodation centres. The census was done at night when people were most likely to be at home. It was found that, although the number of residents had been estimated at 10 000, the actual number of people residing in the accommodation centres was around 6000. The reason for this discrepancy was that many people who were present in the camp during the day were actually returning to their villages at night.

Registration

Registration of refugees or displaced people when they arrive at a site can provide an opportunity to collect data about population size (and structure). Registration can also be combined with other activities, such as distribution of food cards, detection of malnutrition and vaccination against measles.

---

[1] Grais et al. (2005).
[2] Source: Noji (2005).

Data from programme activities

Information from programme activities, such as a vaccine coverage survey of a specific age group (e.g. children aged 6–59 months), can be used to estimate the number of children in this age group as well as the total population.

> For example:
>
> A measles vaccination survey estimates vaccination coverage among children aged 6–59 months in a camp to be 80% (0.8) and 5000 measles vaccines were administered in this age group. Using these data, the number of children aged 6–59 months can be estimated: 5000/0.8 = 6250. If, from another survey, it is known that children in this age group represent 20% of the population in question, the total population can be estimated: 6250/0.2 = 31 250.

Population structure

Since vulnerable groups need to be monitored, it is useful to know what proportion of the population are pregnant women and children under five. The usual methods for determining the population structure include estimation based on the normal distribution of age groups in the general population (see Table 3.1).

Table 3.1 **Distribution standard by age of stable populations in developing countries**

Age group	Proportion of total population
0–4 years	17%
5–14 years	28%
15–29 years	28%
≥30 years	27%
Total	**100%**

However, complex emergencies can affect the normal age and sex structure of populations. For example, there may be proportionally fewer men and proportionally more women, young children and elderly people. It will therefore be necessary to conduct a simple census or sample survey to find out about the age breakdown of the population.

As a minimum it is important to estimate the *expected* number of children under 5 years of age and pregnant women *if the camp population were of the same composition as a normal population.* A quick way to estimate the number of pregnant women is to use the following calculation:

total pregnant women = total population x 0.51 x 0.50 x 0.20

0.51 = 51% = proportion of women in a population.

0.50 = 50% = proportion of women of childbearing age (15–45 years) among all women in the population

0.20 = 20% = chance of any woman aged 15–45 years being pregnant at a given moment, assuming a total fertility rate per woman of childbearing age of 8.[1]

Retrospective mortality

Retrospective mortality data can help to assess how the current situation compares with the recent situation. This is useful for determining trends and the seriousness of the situation (see Box 3.2 for the threshold of gravity based on mortality rates). Methods for estimating retrospective mortality include sample surveys and counting the number of recent graves.

Box 3.2 **Mortality rates and threshold of gravity**

During an emergency, **mortality rates** are expressed as the number of deaths per 10 000 persons per day, whatever the method of data collection. The **threshold of gravity**[1]:

■ of crude mortality = 1 death/10 000 persons per day
■ of mortality in children under 5 = 2 deaths/10 000 children under 5 per day.

---

[1] MSF (1997).

Retrospective mortality survey

Death – the event being quantified – is relatively rare, and the sample therefore needs to be adequately large. For cluster sampling, 30 clusters of 30 families (approximately 4000 individuals) is an appropriate sample size.

The head of each family surveyed is asked about the occurrence (or not) of death within the household during a defined period of time. To avoid

---

[1] In a given population, the total fertility rate (per women 15–45 years) may be, for example 5. If so, a woman is pregnant 5/30 years (16.7%) for 9/12 months (75%); from this, the chance of any woman aged 15–45 years being pregnant at a given time = 16.7% x 75% = 12.5%. At a total fertility rate of 8 children per woman of 15–45 years, 20% of women of childbearing age can be expected to be pregnant at any given time.

43

recall bias and to limit difficulties in interpreting the results, this period of time should be as short as possible but long enough to allow a sufficient number of "death events" to have occurred.

To calculate the mortality rate in the surveyed population:

- Divide the total number of deaths that have occurred in a sample (numerator) by the total number of surveyed individuals alive plus the number who have died (denominator) during a given period of time.
- Multiply the result by 10 000 and relate it to a period of one day to permit comparisons to be made.

For example:

A survey of 5500 individuals showed that there were 49 deaths during the 28 days preceding the survey. The mortality rate was thus $\{[49/(5500 + 49)] \times 10\,000\} / 28 = 3.2$ deaths/10 000 population per day.

Counting recent graves

In some situations it is possible to count the number of graves dug since the arrival of the refugee or displaced population. Although this method is approximate, it provides some useful information when no other data are available.

For example:

Six months after the arrival of a large number of displaced people at Hoddur in Somalia, 5900 graves were counted among a population of 25 000. Thus $5900/(5900 + 25\,000) = 0.19 = 19\%$ of the population died in 6 months, an average of 10.4 deaths/10 000 population per day.

Surveillance priorities in complex emergencies

In an emergency situation:

- Collect only the information that is absolutely necessary.
- Keep data collection as simple as possible.
- Decide who will collect data and from where (see Box 3.3).
- Decide how often to collect information.
- Budget for the costs of surveillance (see Box 3.4).
- Analyse what the information reveals about trends.

Collecting data

In complex emergencies, it is essential to prioritize the surveillance of mortality, the causes of mortality, morbidity, programme effectiveness indicators, and malaria-specific indicators.

Box 3.3 **Collecting data**

Possible approaches to collecting data include involvement of:
- local community health workers working with the team responsible for coordinating health services for the affected population;
- health personnel working in hospitals (outpatient and inpatient departments), health centres, the community, and mobile outreach teams;
- special teams trained to conduct surveys.

Box 3.4 **Budgeting for surveillance**

Human resources
Usually a combination of local and health ministry resources, e.g. vector control teams from the national malaria control programme, reinforced by expatriates. The minimum requirement is one epidemiologist and one laboratory technician. Outreach teams may also be needed, as may additional medical and technical staff to expand services to cope with an increased caseload, and community mobilizers and educators to encourage preventive and early treatment-seeking behaviour.

Laboratory
Costs will depend on whether or not RDTs are used. Other essential laboratory equipment and supplies (see Chapter 5) need to be costed.

Transport
Requirements and costs will depend on the terrain and the accessibility of different areas.

Other costs
Could include forms, equipment or materials required for analysing data, communication equipment, training and administration.

Mortality

Monitoring mortality is essential: death rates are high in the acute phase of an emergency and the immediate priority is to reduce mortality as quickly as possible. Mortality should be assessed across a standardized age group and among pregnant women.

Indicators used for mortality surveillance include:

— number of deaths per 10 000 persons per day: crude mortality rate;
— number of deaths in children under five per 10 000 per day (under-5 mortality rate);
— mortality rate for specific diseases (e.g. malaria, measles, acute respiratory infections, diarrhoea);
— proportion of mortality attributable to specific diseases.

An active mortality surveillance system using home visits should be established and home visitors trained to record total daily deaths and deaths in children under 5 years of age. Each home visitor should cover a population of approximately 1000. Daily data should be compiled and analysed at the end of each week (Table 3.2 provides an example of a surveillance form) together with mortality data from health facilities, to ensure that all available data are included.

Table 3.2 **Example of mortality surveillance form**

Place: ....   Reported by: ....

From:......./......./......... (day/month/year)   To: ..../......./......... (day/month/year)

Population*

Population	End of previous week (A)	New arrivals	Departures	End of this week (B)	Average population (A+B)/2
<5 years old					
All ages					
Pregnant women					

*Information about the population is needed to calculate mortality rate.

Mortality rate

	Number of deaths			Rate (deaths/10 000 per day)		
	Male	Female	Total	Male	Female	Total
<5 years old						
All ages						
Pregnant women						

Causes of mortality

The mortality surveillance system can also be used to collect information about causes of death (Table 3.3 provides an example form). Possible sources of these data include health facility registers, home visits and interviews with household heads. The head of the family is asked about the main symptoms before death. Simple definitions should be used (e.g. for malaria, presence of fever and shivering) and, where feasible, local names. "Closed" questions (requiring Yes or No answers) are preferable for this type of survey.

Table 3.3 **Example form**: **causes of mortality**

Place: .... Reported by: ....

From:....../......./......... (day/month/year) To: ....../......./......... (day/month/year)

Diseases	<5 years of age			≥5 years of age			Total			Percentage
	M	F	Total	M	F	Total	M	F	Total	
Non-bloody diarrhoea										
Bloody diarrhoea										
Severe respiratory infections										
Malaria										
Measles										
Malnutrition										
Suspected meningitis										
War injury										
Others										
Total										

Causes of morbidity

A standardized case definition should be used for each disease, and morbidity should be assessed across a standardized age group and among pregnant women.

Indicators used for morbidity surveillance include:

— incidence rate (the number of new cases per week, expressed as a percentage of the population or per 1000, 10 000 or 100 000 persons).
— incidence rate by age group (e.g. the number of new cases/week in under-fives).

These data can be collected daily from health facilities providing outpatient and inpatient services to the population, and from the community by a mobile team. Daily data should be compiled and analysed at the end of each week.

Programme effectiveness indicators

Information on programme effectiveness indicators should be collected and analysed every week to assess how well different components are functioning.

Indicators that can be used to monitor programme functioning include:

- How many home visitors are working and where?
- How many patients are treated and where?
- How many health personnel are involved?
- What kind of antimalarial drugs are available?
- How long is the delay between ordering the drugs and receiving them into the health facilities?
- Are there frequent shortages of drugs? If so, how long do they last?
- Are rapid diagnostic tests available? Are there frequent shortages of diagnostic supplies? If so, how long do they last?
- What percentage of febrile patients are tested using blood smears or RDTs in outreach activities or in health facilities, and what is the delay (both average and extreme) before test results are known?

Monitoring **case management** is particularly important, to see how well cases are being diagnosed and treated. Indicators that can be used to monitor case management include:

— case-fatality rate (the number of deaths due to a specific disease/total number of cases of the disease per week).

Monitoring **coverage** is also important to ensure that vulnerable groups are being reached or have access to services. Indicators that can be used to assess coverage include:

— the proportion of sick patients with access to a health centre;
— the proportion of affected geographical areas covered by the programme;
— the proportion of pregnant women and under fives covered by the programme.

Malaria-specific indicators

Malaria surveillance should include the indicators summarized in Table 3.4.

Data collected should be based on the standardized WHO definitions (see Box 3.5). Standard case definitions and proper confirmation of cases are essential for accurate surveillance and to make informed judgements about progress. Relying only on clinical diagnosis is likely to provide inaccurate data about malaria cases, so it is important to use a suitable confirmatory tool, such as RDTs or microscopy. Accurate surveillance also depends on good reporting and analysis of data collected.

Table 3.4 **Indicators for malaria surveillance**

Rates	Calculation	Interpretation and decisions
Specific malaria mortality	Number of malaria deaths/ 10 000 per day in each area	Is malaria a health priority?
Proportion of mortality caused by malaria	Number of malaria deaths/ total number of deaths	Is malaria a health priority in the emergency context?
Malaria incidence rate	Number of new malaria cases/total population per week in each area	Is malaria increasing? What action should be taken?
Case-fatality rate in all malaria cases	Number of confirmed malaria deaths/total number of confirmed malaria cases per week in each area	Are cases being managed effectively?
Case-fatality rate in severe malaria cases	Number of confirmed malaria deaths/total number of severe malaria cases	How effective is the referral system and hospital management of cases?
Slide positivity rate	Ratio between the number of confirmed cases and of clinically suspected cases	How good is detection of patients with malaria? Increasing rate may indicate the beginning of a malaria epidemic or a seasonal peak
Proportion of fever caused by malaria	Number of fever cases with confirmed parasitaemia/ total number of fevers	How important a health priority is malaria?

The type of surveillance that is feasible will depend on the phase of the emergency. As discussed in Chapter 2, during a first assessment in the acute phase, surveillance may focus on cross-sectional population surveys to assess the prevalence of disease, or on compiling hospital inpatient data to assess the ratio of malaria to other life-threatening diseases. A malaria survey may be carried out, covering fever incidence, malaria incidence, slide positivity rate and spleen rate. Once the situation stabilizes, however, and microscopy is established, slide positivity rates, RDT positivity rates or malaria incidence rates may be used to guide prioritization of settlements for vector control. For example, in the Afghan refugee camps in Pakistan, only those where incidence exceeded a certain threshold were targeted for vector control. Using this system, preventive interventions were limited to the most endemic camps.

Box 3.5 **Standardized malaria case definitions and classification**[1]

Confirmed uncomplicated malaria

A patient with symptoms and/or signs of malaria, with laboratory confirmation of parasitaemia.

Confirmed severe malaria

A patient who requires hospitalization for symptoms and/or signs of severe malaria, with laboratory confirmation of parasitaemia.

Note: The uncomplicated and severe malaria categories are intended to be mutually exclusive. For example, a patient who initially presents with uncomplicated malaria but then develops signs or symptoms of severe disease should be classified only as having severe malaria, and not counted twice. This also applies to situations where health services record cases as "suspected malaria" until diagnosis is confirmed by microscopy or RDT, after which the cases become "confirmed malaria". Suspected and confirmed malaria cases should be reported separately.

Treatment failure

A patient with treated confirmed malaria who returns with sign and symptoms of malaria and is laboratory confirmed as being parasite-positive within 2–4 weeks of treatment.

Note: Collecting data about patients who return can help to identify problems, for example drug resistance, poor treatment adherence or inadequate diagnosis.

Suspected malaria death

Death of a patient who has been diagnosed with probable severe malaria, with no laboratory confirmation of parasitaemia.

Confirmed malaria death

Death of a patient who has been diagnosed with severe malaria, with laboratory confirmation of parasitaemia.

---

[1] Adapted from: WHO (2000).

Establishing accurate surveillance requires the setting up of microscopy quality control: the service can be provided by technicians of a central reference laboratory who regularly monitor the technical accuracy of microscopists working in field laboratories and clinics. In the Afghan refugee programme, for example, two reference laboratories monitored 45 field laboratories which, in turn, monitored more than 200 camp clinics.

Resistance surveillance

If possible, it is very useful to identify at least one "sentinel site" in a health facility for conducting in vivo resistance surveillance (see Chapter 8). The WHO protocol for in vivo resistance surveillance recommends that a blood smear be carried out for each confirmed malaria patient on days 0, 1, 2, 3, 7, 14 and 28. Resistance surveillance allows the efficacy of first-line treatment to be confirmed and monitored.

Summary

Strategies for establishing an accurate and reliable surveillance system include:

- *Liaison with local health authorities and emergency partners.* Ensure that there is coordination. It can be useful to assign responsibility for organizing and supervising the surveillance system and for coordination to one agency or organization. Integrate the system into the national system as far as possible.

- *Use of standardized case definitions.* Focus on the most significant priority diseases, especially those most likely to cause outbreaks, and provide appropriate training for health workers and staff working for emergency partners.

- *Ensuring that malaria surveillance includes pregnant women.*

- *Rapid re-establishment of laboratory facilities* with confirmatory diagnostic tools (RDTs or microscopy). Provide appropriate training for health workers and laboratory technicians.

- *Re-establishment of a reporting and analysis system.* Set up standardized mechanisms among all emergency partners, provide training, ensure that health workers receive feedback, and support communication between field and district levels.

- *Ensuring that all health facilities are included in the system.* If necessary, set up mobile clinics to provide better coverage of the affected population.

- *Adaptation of reporting frequency to the situation.* Initially – during the acute phase of an emergency – data should be collected weekly. Subsequently this can be done less frequently, e.g. monthly.

References

Grais R et al. (2005). *Are rapid population estimates accurate? A field validation of two different rapid population assessment methods* (in press).

Médecins Sans Frontières (1997). *Refugee health: an approach to emergency situations*. London, Macmillan.

MSF (2005). *Rapid health assessment of refugee or displaced populations*. Médecins Sans Frontières (in press).

Noji EK (2005). Estimating population size in emergencies. *Bulletin of the World Health Organization*, 83(3):164.

WHO (2000). *WHO Expert Committee on Malaria. Twentieth report*. Geneva, World Health Organization (WHO Technical Report Series, No. 892).

CHAPTER 4

Outbreak preparedness and response

This chapter:
- provides guidelines for investigating a malaria outbreak
- describes how to prepare for and respond to an outbreak.

In complex emergencies there are rarely any clearly defined thresholds (mortality or morbidity rates) for a malaria outbreak, but unusual or sudden increases – compared with previous weeks – in malaria mortality, proportional mortality or incidence rates may suggest an outbreak. It is also important to be aware that:

— malaria outbreaks may go on for longer than other disease outbreaks, and can last 3–4 months or even longer depending on the climatic conditions;

— malaria outbreaks often have multiple underlying causes.

In stable situations, an epidemic threshold can be calculated using 5 years' historical data. In a complex emergency it is unlikely that there are sufficient historical data to be useful – unless the camp or settlement area has been established for a long time and accurate malaria data have been collected at least monthly and consistently for several years, allowing comparisons to be made with deviations from the mean or median.

Epidemic malaria may occur in areas of normally low and seasonal malaria transmission where people have little immunity to the disease. It may also occur in non-immune populations who have moved through or into endemic areas. In these cases, severe disease and death due to malaria can occur in all age groups; young children, pregnant women, malnourished individuals and people with concurrent infections (including HIV) are the most vulnerable. Even when malaria transmission is not excessive compared with previous years, local epidemics with high mortality may occur among vulnerable displaced populations because of the concentration of people, the lack of adequate housing and preventive measures (resulting in increased exposure to mosquito bites), concurrent infections and malnutrition, and reduced access to effective treatment.

In the absence of historical data but where recent weekly patient data are available, clear indications of epidemic malaria are a rising slide positivity rate (i.e. increasing numbers of patients with fever have malaria) combined with a rise in the case-fatality rate (non-immune people can die of malaria in a matter of hours, even in well-equipped facilities). Where no comparative data at all are available, a cluster of severe cases and deaths due to febrile disease warrants investigation.

Investigating an outbreak

A suspected malaria outbreak should be investigated immediately, as early intervention is critical. The purpose of an investigation is to:

— confirm the cause of the outbreak with one or more rapid prevalence surveys (high slide positivity rate or rapid diagnosis positivity rate among "fever cases" – see Chapter 2);
— describe the outbreak (age groups, time and geographical distributions, epidemic curve).

Describing the outbreak

Describing the outbreak and planning an effective response require the following:

• Analysis of information from a rapid prevalence survey or surveys.
• Analysis of data collected through the surveillance system, including:
  — retrospective data from registers (if any);
  — prospective data collected using a malaria outbreak form (see Table 4.1); the data should be stratified by population structure (age group, pregnant women) and geographical area (village, district, camp) so that the attack rate can be calculated for different groups and areas and interventions can be targeted to the most vulnerable groups;
  — epidemic curve, which shows graphically (see Figure 4.1) the number of new cases per week and the evolution of the outbreak; regularly updated, the curve can show the transmission season, whether the epidemic has reached its peak, and whether preventive interventions are leading to a reduction in new cases (although variations in access to treatment may make interpretation difficult).

Table 4.1 **Example of malaria outbreak form**

Place: .... Reported by: ....

From:......./......./......... (day/month/year) To: ..../......./......... (day/month/year)

Case definition "malaria" and "malaria death":

_____

_____

Date	Day	New malaria cases				New malaria deaths			
		<5 years	≥5 years	Pregnant women	Total	<5 years	≥5 years	Pregnant women	Total
	1								
	2								
	3								
	4								
	5								
	6								
	7								
Total									

Daily mortality rate (number of "malaria" deaths/10 000 population per day): ....

Weekly attack rate (number of "malaria" cases/1000 population per week): ....

Weekly case-fatality rate (number of "malaria" deaths/number of "malaria" cases x 100): ....

Geographical areas affected (e.g. villages, districts, camps where malaria patients are currently living):

_____

_____

Locality	Estimated total pop. in locality	No. of malaria cases from locality (specify day, week, time period)	No. of malaria deaths from locality (specify day, week, time period)

Comments:

_____

_____

_____

Figure 4.1 **Malaria attack rate (cases/1000 population per week), MSF mobile clinics, Wajir, Kenya, 14 February 1998–19 April 1998**

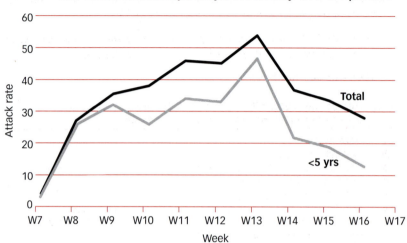

Outbreak preparedness

Measures for epidemic prevention and control can be implemented effectively only if they are supported by an infrastructure of well-trained personnel, adequate supplies and equipment, supervision and evaluation. In areas and populations prone to epidemic malaria, it is essential for partners to agree on and put in place a preparedness plan of action covering the following elements:

- *Supplies* – sufficient stock of essential laboratory diagnosis and treatment supplies for uncomplicated and severe malaria, including rapid diagnostic tests (see Chapter 5); and of equipment, materials, protective clothing and insecticide for emergency prevention activities (see Chapter 6).

- *Laboratory facilities* – an identified laboratory that can determine parasite species and density, and ensure safe blood transfusions.

- *Staff and transport* – staff and transport for mobile teams; the capacity to expand inpatient and outpatient care facilities, including the number of skilled medical and technical staff needed in these facilities (see Box 4.1) to cope with an increased malaria caseload; and the capacity to improve transport and logistics for referral of severe cases to inpatient facilities.

- *Educational messages* – messages to encourage the population to take preventive measures and seek early treatment, and the materials and equipment to get these messages across to the public.

- *Training and refresher training of staff* – on malaria diagnosis, case management, vector control, weekly disease surveillance.

- *Budget* – for all the above.

BOX 4.1 **Medical support staff required – in addition to a doctor – per site dealing with a major malaria epidemic**

- 1 triage nurse
- 1 registration nurse
- 2 nurses for temperature and weight
- 1 person to perform the RDTs
- 2 nurses for dispensing drugs
- 2 nurses for case management of uncomplicated malaria cases
- 24-hour coverage by 1 advanced nurse for care of severe malaria cases
- 1 person for epidemiological surveillance
- 1 driver (to transport referrals)
- 2 health promoters to inform and educate the population.

Outbreak response and follow-up

Coordinate planning and implementation

If there is a confirmed outbreak, all partners – government departments, United Nations agencies, humanitarian aid organizations and NGOs – need to:

- *Decide together how to tackle the outbreak.* Even if the actions of individual players will be limited to certain areas or population groups or focus only on certain methods (e.g. surveillance, disease management/ prevention), it is essential that those actions be coordinated to maximize the impact of interventions. Coordination is especially important if the response involves multiple interventions including, for example, expanding inpatient capacity at referral facilities.

- *Follow good planning principles* – in particular ascertaining which geographical areas and population groups are most affected.

Decide on a strategy

The first priority in an epidemic is prompt and effective diagnosis and treatment with artemisinin-based combination therapy (ACT) for all those who are sick.

Vector control – if well planned, targeted and timely – can contribute significantly to reducing the risk of infection and saving lives. Vector control is most cost-effective when it is implemented for prevention before an epidemic or for control at the very start of an epidemic, i.e. when it is implemented well before the epidemic peak and its subsequent natural decline. High coverage is essential to achieve a "mass effect" and impact on transmission. However, the response to the epidemic is usually delayed and occurs in the middle of the epidemic, with the result that vector control is logistically demanding and time-consuming and its effect is poor.

Vector control interventions should never interfere with, or drain resources from the provision of life-saving treatment to all malaria cases.

The operational strategy for provision of disease management – for example, whether to use mobile teams or (additional) fixed units, whether to focus initially on improvement of inpatient and/or on outpatient care – will depend on:

— the population affected and risk groups (during an outbreak, all age groups may be affected);
— the malaria proportional mortality rate;
— the case-fatality rate;
— the prevalence in different areas;
— access to the existing health facilities – distance to reach health facilities.

A checklist for effective response to malaria epidemics is provided in Annex VIII.

Treatment

It is critical to ensure that there are sufficient treatment points to allow the population to access treatment easily, and that these are providing effective diagnosis and case management. It is also important to ensure that the most vulnerable groups have access to treatment (see Chapters 1 and 2).

Treat positive individuals – treat fever cases

In an outbreak, everyone with a positive parasitaemia result for malaria should be treated immediately, regardless of his or her symptoms. Priority should be given to pregnant women and children under five because they are at particularly high risk of severe disease and death.

In a large epidemic it would be logistically impossible to confirm each case by RDT or microscopy. Therefore, once malaria has been established as the cause of the epidemic (through an RDT survey) and agreement has been reached on a clinical case definition of malaria, mass treatment of malaria/fever cases with ACT is appropriate as a strategy for reducing mortality.

RDTs should be performed on a proportion of patients to track the test positivity rate and the evolution of the epidemic. To ascertain whether the epidemic is still going on and to avoid over-treating, it is useful to carry out RDT surveys among the patients in the waiting room of the health centre at intervals of 2–3 weeks or to make daily RDT checks of a percentage of fever patients.

In an outbreak, pre-referral treatment of severe cases can be improved by using artesunate suppositories to cover the period of transport to a hospital. Rectal artesunate is as effective as quinine during the first 24 hours; to date, however, there is little evidence of its use in the field. If there is a high caseload of severe cases in inpatient facilities, management can be simplified by using IM artemether (see Chapter 5 for more information about treatment and case management).

Prevention

During a malaria outbreak, preventing new cases is also important – but difficult to achieve. The principal interventions to reduce the risk of infection are:

- indoor residual spraying (IRS)
- insecticide-treated nets (ITNs) or other insecticide-treated materials (ITMs).

The most cost-effect interventions are IRS and ITNs if used just before an epidemic or at the very start of an epidemic – that is, applied well before the epidemic peak and its subsequent natural decline. Programmes should aim at high coverage to achieve a "mass effect" and impact on transmission: IRS requires coverage of at least 85% of dwellings to be fully effective. Use of ITNs provides community vector control if population coverage of at least 60% can be achieved (although some studies indicate a figure of 50%): at lower coverage rates, ITNs provide protection only for the people who sleep under them.

Follow-up

Follow-up involves monitoring the evolution of the outbreak and assessing the effectiveness of the response – in terms of how well activities are being carried out, the timing of activities and the level of coverage achieved. Monitoring the impact of interventions is an essential aspect of outbreak follow-up. The evolution of malaria morbidity and mortality over time can be expressed in terms of proportional incidence and case-fatality rates (see Chapter 3).

Repeat prevalence surveys may be needed both to verify whether the outbreak has been brought under control and whenever there are major changes in the composition of the population (e.g. with the arrival of large numbers of non-immune people in endemic areas).

Further reading

WHO (2004). *Malaria epidemics: forecasting, prevention, early detection and control. From policy to practice. Report of an informal consultation, Leysin, Switzerland, 8–10 December 2003.* Geneva, World Health Organization (WHO/HTM/MAL/2004.1098).
- The report summarizes current knowledge and WHO guidance on prevention and control of malaria epidemics. View/download the document at www.who.int/malaria/epidemicstechnicalnorms.html

Hook C (2004). *Field guide for malaria epidemic assessment and reporting: draft for field testing.* Geneva, World Health Organization (WHO/HTM/MAL/2004.1097).
- This guide is written to help field health staff at district and provincial levels to identify malaria epidemics as early as possible after their emergence, and to gather the appropriate information to guide the response. Also:
- *Data entry sheet – epidemic threshold calculation based on 5 years' monthly data –* for use with the above document.
- View/download these documents at www.who.int/malaria/epidemicseds.html

WHO (2002). *Prevention and control of malaria epidemics: 3rd meeting of the Technical Support Network.* Geneva, World Health Organization (WHO/CDS/RBM/2002.40)
- View/download the document at www.who.int/malaria/epidemicstechnicalnorms

CHAPTER 5

Case management

This chapter:

■ provides guidelines for initial management, including *emergency triage* – for the rapid identification and treatment of patients at greatest risk of dying – and *clinical assessment*

■ discusses confirmatory diagnosis of malaria using microscopy and rapid diagnostic tests (RDTs)

■ outlines factors that determine the choice of antimalarial drug

■ describes antimalarial drug treatment for uncomplicated malaria, subsequent follow-up, and the management of treatment failures

■ describes the assessment and treatment of anaemia

■ describes the treatment of severe *P. falciparum* malaria and its associated complications, including resuscitation, treatment with antimalarial drugs, and nursing care

■ provides guidance on the prevention and treatment of malaria in special groups (pregnant women, malnourished patients, returning refugees and displaced persons).

Initial assessment

Emergency triage

Severe malaria is a medical emergency, and patients need to be admitted for immediate treatment and good-quality nursing care. The risk of developing severe malaria depends on the age and immunity of the patient (see Box 5.1).

Many deaths during the acute phase of emergencies can be avoided with prompt identification and effective treatment of all patients who are severely ill (as a result of malaria or any other condition). However, this is not easy in situations where there are few skilled staff and where health facilities are limited and case-loads excessive. It is therefore essential to adopt an emergency triage procedure that is both effective at identifying high-risk patients and simple and quick to perform: the procedure described in

Box 5.1 **Groups at high risk of developing severe malaria**

In all areas:
- pregnant women
- young children
- severely malnourished children and adults (<70% median weight-for-height, or <-3SD[1]).

In areas of high transmission:
- young children
- people of all ages who have been displaced from low-transmission areas and who have little or no immunity.

In areas of low to medium transmission:
- people of all ages with little or no immunity, particularly during outbreaks.

[1] SD = standard deviation score or Z-score. A weight-for-height of −2SD indicates the child is at the lower end of the normal range, and <−3SD indicates severe wasting. A weight-for-height of −3SD is approximately equivalent to 70% of the weight-for-height of the average (median) child. (Source and reference values: http://www.who.int/child-adolescent-health/publications/referral_care/chap7/chap7fr.htm.)

Box 5.2 can identify, in less than 2 minutes, those who need immediate assessment and treatment (see Table 5.1).

Clinical assessment

In complex emergencies in malaria-endemic countries, malaria is responsible for a large proportion of febrile disease, particularly in children. If patients with *P. falciparum* malaria do not receive appropriate treatment with an effective antimalarial drug, they may deteriorate and develop severe malaria within a few hours or days. However, it is important to remember that the clinical presentation of both uncomplicated and severe malaria is variable and nonspecific (see Box 5.3), so that the differential diagnosis of malaria from other febrile illnesses may be difficult. In addition, patients often have more than one underlying disease (for example malaria and meningitis, or malaria and pneumonia). Every effort must be made to improve the capacity to diagnose febrile illnesses by confirmation of the presence of parasites. When this is not feasible, particularly in the acute stages of complex emergencies, the only practical approach may be to treat febrile patients for all suspected diseases with the inevitable consequence that there will be over-treatment not only of malaria but also of other diseases. Knowledge of local disease epidemiology helps in determining the likelihood that any serious illness is due to *P. falciparum*.

Box 5.2 **Danger signs**

Patients with any of the following features need urgent clinical assessment and treatment:

Witnessed convulsions
Convulsions are particularly common in febrile children. Any convulsion that lasts more than 5 minutes requires prompt treatment with diazepam (see "Management of the complications of severe malaria"). Convulsions may present in a subtle way, and important signs include intermittent nystagmus (rapid, jerky eye movements), salivation, and minor twitching of a single finger or toe or of the corner of the mouth.

Prostration
This is:
- the inability to sit unsupported (if aged ≥1 year) *or*
- the inability to drink or breastfeed (if aged <1 year).
Note: Prostration should be actively tested – it is not enough to ask the caregiver.

Coma
This is:
- the inability to localize a painful stimulus[1] (if aged ≥8 months) *or*
- the inability to fix or follow objects with the eyes (if aged 2–8 months[2]).

Respiratory distress
This is deep breathing and/or indrawing of the lower chest wall.
Note: Clothing should be removed so that the breathing pattern can be observed.

[1] Rub firmly on the patient's sternum with the knuckles of one hand. A patient who is able to localize pain will attempt to remove the examiner's hand.

[2] Babies are unable to fix until the age of about 8 weeks.

Although none of the clinical signs listed in Box 5.3 is unique to malaria, those related to severe malaria are a clear indication that a patient is seriously ill and needs immediate investigation and treatment (see Table 5.1 and "Management of severe *P. falciparum* malaria" below).

Confirmatory diagnosis of malaria

Diagnosing malaria on the basis of clinical features alone can be very inaccurate and is likely to result in significant over-treatment or under-treatment of the disease. It is therefore important to establish, at the start of an emergency intervention, the capacity for confirmatory diagnosis.

Table 5.1 **Assessment and treatment of danger signs**

Signs	Check	If:	Treatment[a]
Convulsions	*Duration*	Lasts >5 minutes	Diazepam IV or per rectum
	Blood glucose	<2.2 mmol/l or test not possible	Give 50% dextrose IV
	Malaria slide or RDT	Positive or test not possible	Start antimalarial drugs
	Lumbar puncture (LP)[b]	CSF evidence of meningitis[c] or LP not possible	Start antibiotics for meningitis
Prostration	*Circulation* Capillary refill >3 seconds[d] Weak, fast pulse Cold hands	Any sign positive (indicates shock) and no evidence of severe malnutrition	Start rapid IV fluids Give oxygen
	Hydration Sunken eyes Lax skin turgor[e]	Any sign positive (indicates dehydration) and no evidence of severe malnutrition	Start rapid IV fluids or insert nasogastric (NG) tube and start oral rehydration solution
	Nutrition Visible severe wasting AND/OR Flaking skin and oedema of both feet	Any sign positive (indicates severe malnutrition)	Transfer to therapeutic feeding centre
	Blood glucose	<2.2 mmol/l or test not possible	Give 50% dextrose IV
	Lumbar puncture If none of the above signs is present, perform LP	CSF evidence of meningitis[c] or LP not possible	Start antibiotics for meningitis
	Malaria slide or RDT	Positive or test not possible	Start antimalarials
Coma	*Blood glucose*	<2.2 mmol/l or test not possible	Give dextrose 50% IV
	Perform LP	CSF evidence of meningitis[c] or LP not possible	Start antibiotics for meningitis
	Malaria slide or RDT	Positive[f] or test not possible	Start IV or IM antimalarials
	All comatose patients		Insert NG tube, aspirate stomach contents

Table 5.1 *Continued*

Signs	Check	If:	Treatment[a]
	Palmar pallor Check Hb	Hb <5g/dl	Give immediate blood transfusion
Respiratory distress	*Hydration* Lethargy Sunken eyes Lax skin turgor[e]	Any sign positive and no evidence of severe malnutrition	Start rapid IV fluids
	Circulation Capillary refill >3 seconds Weak, fast pulse Cold hands	Any sign positive and no evidence of severe malnutrition	Insert IV and start rapid IV fluids
	Listen to chest	Chest crackles	Verify pulmonary oedema;[g] start anti-biotics for pneumonia

[a] For treatment details see "Management of severe *P. falciparum* malaria", page 85.

[b] Lumbar puncture should be performed if the patient is still unconscious more than 30 minutes after the end of a convulsion.

[c] CSF evidence of meningitis: CSF: blood glucose ratio <0.5, CSF protein >0.6 g/litre, bacteria seen on Gram stain. When measurement of glucose and protein is not possible, cloudy CSF should be taken as indicative of meningitis.

[d] Capillary refill: apply pressure for 3 seconds to whiten the fingernail; determine the capillary refill time from the moment of release to recovery of original nail colour.

[e] Skin turgor: pinch the skin of abdomen halfway between the umbilicus and the side for 1 second, then release and observe; if the skin takes >2 seconds to return, this indicates dehydration.

[f] In all cases of suspected severe malaria, parenteral antimalarial chemotherapy must be started immediately. If the cause of coma is in doubt, also test for (and treat) other locally prevalent causes of coma, e.g. bacterial, fungal or viral meningoencephalitis. If the malaria slide/RDT is negative it must be repeated, and the Giemsa-stained slide must be examined for indirect signs of parasitaemia (pigment in neutrophils).

[g] If pulmonary oedema is suspected, position the patient upright, give oxygen, stop IV fluids and give frusemide, 1 mg/kg IV. If pulmonary oedema is associated with blood transfusion, give frusemide, 1 mg/kg IV, and restart transfusion at a slower rate.

Box 5.3 **Clinical features of uncomplicated and severe malaria**

Uncomplicated malaria	Severe malaria
Clinical features of uncomplicated malaria may include:	A patient with severe falciparum malaria may present with confusion or drowsiness with extreme weakness (prostration). In addition, the following may develop:
Fever	
Headache	Cerebral malaria, defined as unrousable
Vomiting	coma not attributable to any other cause
Diarrhoea	in a patient with falciparum malaria
Cough	Generalized convulsions
Influenza-like symptoms,	Severe normocytic anaemia
e.g. chills, muscle pains	Hypoglycaemia
Febrile convulsions	Metabolic acidosis with respiratory distress
(in children)	Fluid and electrolyte disturbances
	Acute renal failure
	Acute pulmonary oedema and adult respiratory distress syndrome (ARDS)
	Circulatory collapse, shock, septicaemia ("algid malaria")
	Abnormal bleeding (bruising, bleeding gums)
	Jaundice
	Haemoglobinuria secondary to haemolysis
	High fever
	Hyperparasitaemia

Important: These severe manifestations can occur singly or, more commonly, in combination in the same patient.

Effective confirmatory diagnosis can help to:
— identify patients who need antimalarial treatment;
— reduce unnecessary use of antimalarial drugs for patients without malaria;
— identify malaria species;
— identify treatment failures.

The need for parasitological confirmation of diagnosis in individual patient management depends on the level of transmission and the age of the patient. Laboratory confirmation is needed for:

— all patients with suspected malaria in areas of low to moderate transmission;
— all adults and all children aged 5 years and over with suspected malaria in areas of high transmission.

Laboratory confirmation is not strictly needed for:

— children under 5 years of age with suspected malaria in high-transmission areas; these children can be treated on the basis of clinical diagnosis (fever) alone, following the IMCI algorithm, bearing in mind that a child's illness may commonly have more than one pathological basis and that fever does not necessarily mean malaria, even in high-transmission areas;

— every single fever patient once malaria has been established as the cause of an ongoing epidemic with massive case-loads that overwhelm the health services.

- *In areas of low transmission and during epidemics*, where populations have little immunity to malaria, malaria infection is dangerous for all age groups. The presence of malaria parasites in the peripheral blood (detected by confirmatory diagnosis) almost always indicates that the patient has, or will develop, clinical malaria and therefore requires treatment.

- *In areas of stable moderate to high transmission*, which include large parts of sub-Saharan Africa, people who have been regularly exposed to malaria since infancy have usually developed partial immunity. Where transmission is perennially high, a large proportion of the population may have malaria parasites in their blood, yet relatively few of them will become ill.

There are two options for confirmatory diagnosis of malaria:

— light microscopy
— rapid diagnostic tests (RDTs).

The characteristics and potential uses of these two methods are outlined below.

Light microscopy
Performance
Microscopy is the "gold standard" and the most commonly used laboratory diagnostic tool in malaria-endemic regions. When performed by a skilled technician, microscopy is more sensitive than RDTs for the detection of low levels of *P. falciparum* parasitaemia (<100 parasites/µl) and can differentiate between the various malaria species. When poorly performed, however, microscopy produces unreliable results.

Effective microscopy for malaria parasites requires good quality equipment and reagents, skilled technicians who can prepare and stain films, identify parasites, and differentiate between *Plasmodium* species, and rigorous technical supervision and quality control. However, since these may not be available in complex emergency situations, it is often necessary for emergency partners to establish the capacity themselves. This requires training, investment in equipment (basic binocular microscopes that do not require electricity, or that can operate using electricity or natural light are the most appropriate option), and budgeting for recurrent costs, such as reagents. Once established, the direct cost of microscopy ranges from US$ 0.12–0.40 per test.

When to use microscopy

- *Routine confirmatory diagnosis and patient management.* Microscopy services, including training and supervision, should be re-established as an emergency situation stabilizes and used for routine confirmation of malaria and for management of severe malaria.

- *Investigation of suspected treatment failures.* Microscopic examination of thick and thin peripheral blood films should be carried out to confirm all cases of suspected treatment failure.

- *Drug efficacy studies.* Microscopy should be used for studies that assess the therapeutic efficacy of antimalarial drugs.

- *Quality control system for rapid diagnostic tests.* Quality control of RDTs in the field is needed to verify both batch quality and possible deterioration of quality during transport and storage. At least one reference laboratory is needed for verification of RDT results against good microscopy, with a small percentage of RDTs being regularly compared.

Rapid diagnostic tests
Design
Rapid diagnostic tests (RDTs) for malaria use a dipstick, cassette or test card designed to detect malaria parasite antigens in the blood of an infected individual. The main types of commercially available RDT detect:

- — histidine-rich protein II (HRP-II), a water-soluble protein produced only by *P. falciparum*;
- — HRP-II plus a nonspecific pan-malaria antigen (detects all four malaria species);
- — lactate dehydrogenase (pLDH), *P. falciparum*-specific and pan-specific.

HRP-II kits detect only *P. falciparum*. Kits combining HRP-II and a pan-malarial antigen, as well as pLDH kits, can distinguish *P. falciparum* from non-falciparum species, but cannot distinguish between *P. vivax*, *P. ovale* and *P. malariae*, or between *P. falciparum* alone and a mixed *P. falciparum*/non-falciparum infection. A few recently released products can also distinguish *P. vivax* from other species.

Performance

Accuracy in the detection of P. falciparum

Initial evaluation of their performance in different epidemiological and clinical settings showed that, at parasite densities above 100/µl blood, RDTs can detect *P. falciparum* with >90% sensitivity of. That is, more than 90% of cases with malaria parasitaemia test positive on RDT, which is equivalent to the sensitivity that can normally be achieved with skilled microscopy. In cases with parasite densities below 100/µl blood, RDT sensitivity decreases markedly.

More recent reports, however, have indicated sensitivities and specificities for *P. falciparum* well below those required for operational use. It is thought that problems with storage and transport and a lack of quality control may have contributed to these results, which emphasize the need to ensure good quality assurance for RDTs and continued monitoring of their efficacy.

Mixed species infections

In areas where two or more *Plasmodium* species commonly occur together, patients may present with mixed malaria infections. RDT kits sensitive to both *P. falciparum* and non-falciparum species cannot simultaneously demonstrate the presence of more than one species and are designed to detect *P. falciparum* preferentially. In the absence of *P. falciparum*, these test kits will show infection by a non-falciparum species, although their sensitivity in detecting *P. vivax* is low, especially with low parasitaemia.

Storage and transport

Most RDT products should be stored and transported within the temperature range 4–30 °C, which is most likely to be impossible in many of the situations where they are used operationally. RDTs are sensitive to both moisture (humidity) and high temperatures. Where they are used, storage and transport conditions should be carefully controlled and documented.

Relative cost

In practical terms, the overall cost of using RDTs – which includes organization, personnel, supervision and quality control – is likely to be lower than that of maintaining reliable, high-quality microscopy if microscopic diagnosis is used only infrequently.

Box 5.4 summarizes the advantages of RDTs in emergency situations.

Box 5.4 **Advantages of rapid diagnostic tests in emergency situations**

Rapid diagnostic tests:
— are quick to perform (in practice, about 20 minutes for most tests)
— if of good quality, produce reliable results
— are sensitive on detecting *P. falciparum*, which causes severe malaria
— do not need skilled laboratory technicians, and can be used by health workers and non-health workers after a few hours of training
— do not need electricity or laboratory equipment
— are suitable for diagnosis when case-loads are high – a team of two people can process more than 200 tests a day, making RDTs particularly useful as a screening tool during community surveys
— cost from US$ 0.65 per test for detection of *P. falciparum* and from US$ 1.00 per test for detection of all species (although prices should be checked with individual manufacturers).

When to use RDTs

Confirmatory diagnosis of suspected malaria cases

In low-transmission areas where there are relatively few malaria cases and/or where health staff may not be skilled in malaria microscopy, RDTs provide an effective alternative to microscopy for the diagnosis of malaria, provided that they are of assured quality.

In high-transmission settings, RDTs may be used for confirmation of severe malaria until the situation is stabilized and good-quality microscopy services are established. They can also be used when it is impossible to establish or maintain effective microscopy services as a result, for example, of inadequate resources or the risk of looting.

Rapid malaria assessments

RDTs are particularly useful for screening large numbers of people for malaria, particularly when combined with a record of clinical symptoms (actual or reported fever). They are therefore well suited to malaria surveys/assessments (either community cross-sectional or clinic-based), especially when these must be completed and analysed quickly as part of an emergency assessment, and when the identification of non-falciparum species is not necessary.

Malaria epidemics

In epidemic situations, where patient numbers are very high, RDTs can enable a team of two people to accurately screen up to 200 patients per day. Where this is not possible, because of shortages of either staff or RDTs, clinical diagnosis may be the only option. RDTs can then be used to confirm a proportion of clinically diagnosed cases. In an ongoing malaria epidemic, most fever cases presenting at health facilities will be malaria, and over-treatment of non-malaria cases will be minimal; however, this proportion will fall in the later stages of the epidemic and, if confirmatory diagnostic capacity is not then established, the degree of over-treatment will increase significantly (see Box 5.5).

Box 5.5 **Diagnosing malaria during an epidemic in Burundi**

In late 2000 and early 2001, a malaria epidemic occurred in the highlands of Burundi, an area already affected by a long-term complex emergency. The epidemic threatened 2 million people – about 30% of the population.

Accurate diagnosis of suspected malaria cases was difficult because of the large number of patients. Daily case-loads were as high as 2000 in some clinics. In Kayanza, one of the worst-affected provinces, RDTs were used initially to confirm the epidemic. Since 80% of the people attending the clinics were positive for *P. falciparum*, it was decided to treat patients on the basis of clinical symptoms and to use RDTs on a sample of one in five patients attending for treatment at sentinel sites.

As the epidemic waned, the proportion of parasite-positive patients fell to 40–50% and the need for laboratory confirmation of clinical diagnosis increased. However, this was extremely difficult to implement, because of severe staff shortages and the very high numbers of people attending health facilities.

When not to use RDTs

RDTs that detect HRP-II may continue to produce positive test results for up to 14 days after effective treatment of a malaria infection, even though patients no longer have detectable parasites on microscopy. These tests should therefore not be used for the following purposes.

Investigation of suspected treatment failures

Microscopy should be used to confirm treatment failure. When microscopy is not possible, the decision to give further antimalarial treatment relies upon the history of first-line treatment.

Drug efficacy studies
Microscopy should be used for drug efficacy studies. Microscopy can also provide quantitative results (parasite counts).

Treatment overview
Factors that determine the choice of antimalarial drugs
The choice of drugs to be used for the treatment of malaria will depend on:

— the local parasite species
— the local drug-resistance patterns of the parasites
— high therapeutic efficacy
— acceptable human tolerance (safety)
— good adherence
— availability
— acceptability to patients and to the health authorities
— acceptability of cost to the drug provider.

Therapeutic efficacy
Antimalarial drug resistance, the misuse of drugs, and the use of poor-quality drugs are important causes of treatment failure.

Global malaria control is being threatened on an unprecedented scale by the rapidly growing resistance of *Plasmodium falciparum* to conventional treatments such as chloroquine, sulfadoxine–pyrimethamine (SP) and amodiaquine. Multidrug-resistant falciparum malaria is widely prevalent in south-east Asia and South America. Now Africa, the continent with the highest burden of malaria, is also being seriously affected by drug resistance. Because of the risk of treatment failure due to drug resistance, national antimalarial drug policies normally include at least two lines of treatment of uncomplicated malaria.

Populations in complex emergencies are more vulnerable to malaria disease, and their first-line treatment for falciparum malaria must therefore be of the highest possible efficacy. In these situations, where mortality is high, drug combinations that include an artemisinin derivative are recommended. Current choices of artemisinin-based combination therapy (ACT) are artemether–lumefantrine, artesunate–amodiaquine, artesunate–SP and artesunate–mefloquine. The efficacy of ACT depends on resistance to the artemisinin partner drug. A new ACT chosen as part of local drug policy in a complex emergency should have an efficacy of at least 95%. If no information on local drug efficacy patterns is available in African countries, the choice should be artemether–lumefantrine (Coartem®), which is still >95% efficacious in Africa. In chronic-phase emergencies, 2-yearly therapeutic efficacy testing of ACT should be carried out in sentinel sites to ascertain that it remains above 90%.

Information on antimalarial drug resistance and the testing protocol is available at www.who.int/malaria/resistance.html.

Once the emergency stabilizes, national authorities will be faced with longer-term decisions regarding drug choice, and information gained earlier in the emergency may be very helpful. In countries where monotherapy (e.g. chloroquine, SP) is still used for first- and second-line treatment but where the efficacy of these drugs has been compromised by resistance, WHO recommends changing to ACT as first-line treatment for uncomplicated malaria.

Availability

A coordinated approach is essential if adequate supplies of good quality antimalarial drugs are to be provided on a regular basis. The standardized purchase and supply of recommended, good-quality antimalarial drugs are the responsibility of all emergency partners. WHO – in collaboration with UNICEF – has established a system for pre-qualification of manufacturers of artemisinin derivatives, negotiated price agreements with manufacturers, undertaken international procurement, and set up systems of pharmacovigilance. A broader service for malaria medicines and supplies has been established by the RBM partnership to facilitate access to high-quality, affordable antimalarial medicines and other essential supplies: insecticide-treated mosquito nets, rapid diagnostic tests (RDT), and insecticides. For information and assistance, contact the RBM Malaria Medicines and Supplies Service (MMSS), http://rbm.who.int/mmss.

Operational feasibility

Operational feasibility is determined by patient numbers, resources, and access to health facilities. It is best to use drugs that are effective and simple to administer: for example, once-daily intramuscular artemether is preferable to 8-hourly intravenous infusions of quinine for the treatment of severe malaria.

In emergency situations, limited access to health facilities and poor security may mean that the health worker sees a patient only once. In these circumstances, patient adherence to multi-day therapies may be poor and can lead to treatment failure. It is therefore vital that the treatment regimen is properly explained, both to the clinician (who may be unfamiliar with the recommended therapy) and to each patient.

Management of uncomplicated *P. falciparum* malaria
Supportive and ancillary treatment of young children

When an antimalarial drug is given to a young child, the chance of the child vomiting the medication will be lower if fever (axillary temperature >37.5 °C) is first treated with an antipyretic and with tepid sponging. Antipyretic drugs such as paracetamol or ibuprofen (an expensive but effective alternative to paracetamol) should be used: aspirin is not recommended in children because it can cause a rare but serious condition called Reye syndrome, which affects the liver and the brain.

Children should remain at the clinic for an hour after the first dose of antimalarial drug (see Annex IV for information about the safety of antimalarial drugs in young children). Ideally, outpatient facilities should have a shaded area where patients and carers can wait. Carers should be encouraged to sponge febrile children with tepid water. If it is not possible for a child to wait at the clinic, the parent or carer should be told to return if the child vomits within the first hour; the child should then be re-treated with a full dose of the antimalarial drug. A child who vomits the drug more than once should be admitted as an inpatient. It is important to watch for signs of dehydration and to give appropriate treatment if necessary. Carers should be told that it is important for infants to breastfeed frequently, and for older children to drink plenty of fluid, to prevent dehydration.

Antimalarial drug treatment: choosing the most appropriate drug(s)

WHO recommends that any country experiencing resistance to antimalarial monotherapies should adopt a policy of using combination therapies for first-line treatment of falciparum malaria – preferably those containing an artemisinin derivative.[1] In practice, this applies worldwide with the current exception of Central America, the island of Hispaniola, and those few countries with pure vivax malaria. The increased vulnerability of populations in complex emergencies requires the use of highly effective ACTs even if these are not yet included in routine national treatment policies.

In south-east Asia, ACTs have been shown to improve treatment efficacy and to contain drug resistance.

---

[1] Position of WHO's Roll Back Malaria Department on malaria treatment policy, www.rbm.who.int (accessed September 2005).

The advantages of ACT are:

— rapid reduction of parasite numbers;
— rapid resolution of clinical symptoms;
— effective action against multidrug-resistant *P. falciparum*;
— as yet, no documented resistance to artemisinin and its derivatives;
— few clinical adverse reactions; and
— reduction of gametocyte carriage rates, which reduces patient infec-
tivity to mosquitoes.

Widespread use of ACT as a component of a comprehensive malaria control programme contributes to a reduction in overall malaria transmission.
Experience to date indicates that this effect may be more apparent in areas
of low transmission than in areas of high transmission.

Artesunate is the most commonly used oral formulation of the artemisinin derivatives. Although the price is gradually falling, artesunate remains
expensive compared with the commonly used monotherapies.

Artesunate is highly effective against blood stages of the malaria parasite, but 7 days of treatment are required when it is used as monotherapy – a
3-day regime would result in recrudescence rates of up to 50%. However,
a 3-day course of artesunate combined with another blood schizonticide as
part of ACT is fully effective.

The options for artemisinin-based combination therapy for uncomplicated falciparum malaria are listed in Box 5.6.

Artemisinin-based combination therapy options
Fixed-dose combination
Artemether–lumefantrine (Coartem®)
Artemether–lumefantrine is the only fixed-dose ACT currently available.
To date, clinical trials involving more than 3000 patients, including 600
children under 5 years of age, have been carried out in Africa, south-east
Asia and Europe and show high cure rates and tolerability. The combina-
tion should be taken as a 6-dose regimen.

Artemether–lumefantrine will be the standard antimalarial included in
the upcoming 2005 Inter-Agency Emergency Health Kit – it is particularly
useful in complex emergency situations where there are no local data on the
efficacy of drugs contained in other combination options. It is essential that
Coartem® is taken with fatty food of some kind, such as a glass of milk or
some peanuts.

Box 5.6 **Artemisinin-based combination therapy for uncomplicated falciparum malaria**

Fixed combination treatment
The two drugs are co-formulated in a single tablet:
■ *artemether* plus *lumefantrine* (Coartem®)
■ *dihydro-artemisinin* plus *piperaquine* (Artekin® – in advanced development)
■ *artesunate* plus *mefloquine* (expected in 2006)
■ *artesunate* plus *amodiaquine* (expected in 2006)

Non-fixed combination treatment
The drugs are formulated in separate tablets, which may be combined in a blister pack:
■ *artesunate* (4 mg/kg once a day for 3 days) plus *mefloquine* (25 mg/kg, ideally as a split dose – 15 mg/kg followed after 12–24 hours by 10 mg/kg – to reduce the risk of vomiting, but may be given as a single dose of 25 mg/kg where a split dose is not possible)
■ *artesunate* (4 mg/kg once a day for 3 days) plus *sulfadoxine–pyrimethamine* (SP) (adults: 3 tablets: 1500 mg sulfadoxine + 75 mg pyrimethamine; children: sulfa component 25 mg/kg + pyrimethamine component 1.25 mg/kg, as a single dose on day 1)
■ *artesunate* (4 mg base/kg once a day for 3 days) plus *amodiaquine* (10 mg base/kg daily for 3 days: total dose 30 mg base/kg)

See Annex V for detailed dosage regimens.

Note: Due to limited or non-availability of data, the ACT treatments listed above are not recommended in the first trimester of pregnancy. Nevertheless, ACT treatment should not be withheld if the infection is confirmed and life-threatening and no alternative treatment is available.

Delivery. The absorption of lumefantrine, a hydrophobic, lipophilic compound, is variable and increases when the drug is taken with food (particularly fatty foods). Drug absorption therefore increases as the appetite returns with clinical recovery. Absorption is increased by more than 100% when artemether–lumefantrine is taken with a meal rich in fat. In practice, therefore, the drug combination must be taken with some food. If the patient is too ill to eat, or if field conditions prevent this, a glass of milk or similar drink should be given with each dose until the patient is able to eat normally. (See Annex V for dosage schedule.)

Side-effects. Although the artemether–lumefantrine combination is generally well tolerated, the following side-effects have been reported: dizziness and fatigue, anorexia, nausea, vomiting, abdominal pain, palpitations, myalgia, sleep disorders, arthralgia, headache and rash. The side-effects are generally mild, however, and there is no indication of cardiotoxicity.

Contraindications. Artemether–lumefantrine is contraindicated in:

— persons with known hypersensitivity to either of the component drugs;
— persons with severe malaria.

Safety in special groups. The safety of artemether–lumefantrine has not yet been established in children of less than 5 kg body weight, and its use in this group is not recommended until further safety data are available. Artemether–lumefantrine is not recommended in the first trimester of pregnancy.

Non-fixed-dose combinations

The two drugs – artesunate plus another antimalarial – used in these combinations are separately formulated as tablets.

Because of the rapid development of resistance to SP and cross-resistance between chloroquine and amodiaquine, which is of concern in areas of high chloroquine resistance, it is important to know the therapeutic efficacy of these options before they are introduced. If data are not available from WHO or local experts, or have not already been obtained through operational research, artemether–lumefantrine is likely to be a better option. This can be reviewed once adequate drug efficacy data for other ACT options have been obtained.

Contraindications to artesunate. The following contraindications apply to all the combinations listed below. Artesunate should not be used:

— when there is a history of allergy to artemisinin derivatives;
— for first-line treatment of uncomplicated malaria in the first trimester of pregnancy (but, in areas of multidrug resistance, artemisinin derivatives may be used during the second and third trimesters).

Artesunate plus mefloquine

The combination of artesunate plus mefloquine can be used in areas where *P. falciparum* is resistant to chloroquine, SP and amodiaquine. It also provides an effective alternative to artemether–lumefantrine for emergency situations in which the efficacy of SP and amodiaquine is unknown.

Delivery. Many young children (particularly those aged under 5 years) and older patients with fever vomit the first dose of mefloquine. Vomiting can be reduced if the recommended dose of 25 mg/kg is given as a split dose over 2 days on days 2 and 3 of treatment (15 mg/kg followed 24 hours later by 10 mg/kg). Artesunate is given on days 1, 2 and 3. (See Annex V for dosage schedule.) The absorption of mefloquine is improved when the drug is taken with plenty of water or following food. There should be no re-treatment with mefloquine within 8 weeks of previous treatment. A fixed-dose combination is expected to become available in 2006.

Side-effects. The commonest side-effects of mefloquine are nausea, vomiting, dizziness, sleep disorders, anxiety and other neurological symptoms.

Serious neuropsychiatric adverse reactions have been reported in people treated with mefloquine, including – rarely – psychosis, toxic encephalopathy, convulsions and acute brain syndrome. The frequency of serious side-effects appears to be dose-related, and the risk has been reported to be 7-fold higher among people who have been re-treated with mefloquine within 4 weeks of previous treatment. Mefloquine has been associated with an increased risk of stillbirth in large observational studies in Thailand, but not in Malawi.

Contraindications. Mefloquine should not be used in the following situations:

— when there is a history of allergy to mefloquine;
— when there is a history of severe neuropsychiatric disease;
— in persons who have received mefloquine in the previous 8 weeks;
— during the first trimester of pregnancy (but, in areas of multidrug resistance, mefloquine may be used in combination with artesunate in the second and third trimesters, for example if the risk of malaria is high and there are no alternative efficacious drugs).

Artesunate plus sulfadoxine–pyrimethamine

The combination of artesunate plus SP is an option for use in emergencies in parts of the world where there is good parasite sensitivity to SP. However, most of south-east Asia, some of south America (particularly the Amazon basin), most of east Africa, and increasing areas of central Africa now have significant SP resistance, and reports of resistance in west Africa are increasing. In areas of significant SP resistance, an alternative artemisinin-based combination should be selected. The rapid spread of resistance to SP means that its use as monotherapy and in ACT is now limited.

Delivery. The practical operational advantage of SP over other combination options in that the full dose of SP is delivered as a single dose on day 1 and can be given at the same time as the first dose of artesunate. SP is less likely than mefloquine to cause vomiting in young children. (See Annex V for dosage schedule.) Folic acid, if administered concurrently with SP, may antagonize the action of sulfadoxine; delivery of folic acid supplements should therefore be delayed until 1 week after SP treatment.

Side-effects. SP is generally well tolerated when used as recommended and severe adverse side-effects are rare. However, allergic reactions of varying severity have been reported and are more common after repeated dosing. In practice, patients should not be treated with SP if they have received SP in the previous 4 weeks or if they have known hypersensitivity to sulfa drugs. While cutaneous reactions are quite rare, they are more common in patients who are HIV-positive. This should be taken into account when dealing with known high-risk groups, especially in long-term camp settings where sexual abuse and prostitution may be major issues.

SP should *not* be used for prophylaxis. Severe erythema multiforme involving the skin and mucous membranes (Stevens–Johnson syndrome) and toxic epidermal necrolysis have been reported in between 1 in 5000 and 1 in 8000 people taking SP for weekly chemoprophylaxis.

Contraindications. SP should not be used in the following situations:

— when there is known hypersensitivity to sulfa drugs or pyrimethamine;
— for chemoprophylaxis;
— when there is severe hepatic or renal dysfunction;
— in children under 2 months old;
— in those who have received treatment with SP in the previous 4 weeks.

Artesunate plus amodiaquine

The combination of artesunate plus amodiaquine can be used in all regions where resistance to amodiaquine is still low. In practice this is limited to parts of Africa. Therapeutic efficacy of amodiaquine in areas of chloroquine-resistant malaria may be compromised as a result of cross-resistance and, in the absence of in vivo efficacy data, the therapeutic efficacy of amodiaquine should not be assumed.

Delivery. Amodiaquine tablets are more palatable than chloroquine and are therefore easier to administer to children. Amodiaquine is metabolized rapidly and extensively and does not need to be delivered with food. (See Annex V for dosage schedule.) A fixed-dose artesunate–amodiaquine combination will become available in early 2006.

Side-effects. Standard treatment doses of amodiaquine produce side-effects similar to those observed with chloroquine. These include nausea, vomiting, abdominal pain, diarrhoea and itching; bradycardia is a less common side-effect. Amodiaquine should not be used for chemoprophylaxis, as this may cause life-threatening hepatitis and agranulocytosis.

Contraindications. Amodiaquine should not be used in the following situations:

— when there is known hypersensitivity to amodiaquine;
— in persons with hepatic disorders;
— for chemoprophylaxis.

Follow-up and treatment failures
Immediate follow-up
Carers and/or patients should be instructed to return to the health facility for priority care if a patient repeatedly vomits treatment, has convulsions or becomes increasingly drowsy.

Longer-term follow-up
Carers and/or patients should be instructed to return to the health facility if symptoms worsen or if symptoms have not resolved by day 4 of treatment.

Treatment failures
Definition
Treatment failure is defined as the failure to effectively clear malaria parasites from the blood, with a recurrence of symptoms within days or weeks of the initial antimalarial treatment. The time at which symptoms recur depends partly upon the duration of action of the antimalarial drug. There are several clinical pictures of treatment failure:

— clinical deterioration, which may lead to severe disease;
— slow clinical response;
— apparent resolution of clinical symptoms followed by a reappearance of malaria-related symptoms;
— chronic anaemia secondary to repeated parasitaemic episodes.

Causes
Treatment failure may be caused by any (or a combination) of the following:

- *Vomiting or poor absorption.* The patient or carer may have been confused about what to do when treatment has been vomited or about the need to take Coartem® with some fatty food.

- *Drug quality.* Treatment failure can result from the use of poor-quality or counterfeit antimalarial drugs that do not contain the recommended amount of active ingredient. This is a risk if patients are receiving treatment from poorly-supervised public or private health facilities. The quality of ACTs should be ensured by always obtaining supplies through reputable pharmaceutical companies/agencies – and preferably directly from producers.

- *Poor prescribing practice.* The prescription of an incomplete course of antimalarial treatment increases the risk of treatment failure.

- *Poor adherence.* Poor adherence to treatment may be caused by a number of factors, including the following:
  — The correct regimen may have been unclear to the patient or carer.
  — Patients may choose to stop taking the treatment once initial symptoms have resolved. This is a particular problem with drugs that produce very rapid clearance of symptoms.
  — After taking the initial antimalarial drug dose, a patient may choose to share the remaining treatment with family members.
  — In areas with cost-recovery systems for health care, many patients cannot afford to buy a complete course of treatment. In these circumstances, a health worker whose salary is paid through the cost-recovery system may be tempted to sell patients incomplete courses of treatment.

- *Drug resistance.* Drug resistance is the ability of a parasite to survive and/or multiply despite the administration and absorption of a drug given in doses equal to or higher than those usually recommended (but well within the tolerance of the patient).

The management of suspected treatment failure depends upon the drug that was used for first-line treatment.

- All patients presenting with severe malaria symptoms should be urgently treated with one of the drug therapies recommended in Box 5.9.
- Repeat treatment should be carefully supervised. The following are the treatment options:
  — *Option 1*: artemether–lumefantrine (Coartem®) 6-dose regimen.
  — *Option 2*: 7-day course of oral artesunate (2 mg/kg per day).

— *Option 3*: 7-day course of oral quinine (10 mg of salt/kg 3 times daily).

— *Option 4*: (for areas of multidrug resistance): 7-day course of oral quinine (10 mg of salt/kg 3 times daily) plus 7 days of oral doxycycline (adults: 100 mg daily, with a double dose on the first day) or 7 days of oral clindamycin (5 mg/kg 3 times daily). Doxycycline (but not clindamycin) is contraindicated for pregnant women and children <8 years.

The choice of drug will depend on the antimalarial drug already taken, the availability of alternatives, contraindications for the various medications, and operational feasibility. Adherence to the full course of re-treatment is vital, and re-treatment should be supervised where possible. Adherence to 7-day drug regimens is improved if detailed instructions are given to patients, carers and health personnel.

Management of non-falciparum malaria
Chloroquine

Treatment with chloroquine is the standard recommended therapy for malaria caused by *P. vivax*, *P. malariae* and *P. ovale*. In chloroquine-sensitive areas, a 3-day course of treatment kills most stages of all the non-falciparum species. However, chloroquine does not kill the liver stages (hypnozoites) of *P. vivax* or *P. ovale*, for which an additional drug, primaquine, is required.

Chloroquine resistance and alternative therapy

Chloroquine resistance of *P. vivax* is rare and was first reported in the late 1980s in Indonesia and Papua New Guinea. Focal "true" chloroquine resistance (i.e. in patients with adequate blood levels at day of failure) or prophylactic and/or treatment failure have also been observed in Brazil, Colombia, Ethiopia, Guatemala, Guyana, India, Myanmar, Peru, the Republic of Korea, Solomon Islands, Thailand and Turkey. *P. malariae* resistant to chloroquine has been reported from Indonesia. Treatment options for confirmed chloroquine-resistant vivax malaria include mefloquine, quinine and artesunate (see Box 5.7); SP is not recommended as it is slow to clear vivax parasites.

Anti-relapse treatment for vivax malaria

The standard anti-relapse treatment for the dormant liver stage of *P. vivax* and *P. ovale* is primaquine, 0.5 mg base/kg per day for 14 days in south-

82

Box 5.7 **Oral drug treatment for non-falciparum malaria**

Option 1	chloroquine: base 10 mg/kg once daily for 2 days, then 5 mg/kg on day 3 (in chloroquine-sensitive areas)
Option 2	mefloquine: 15 mg/kg as a single dose
Option 3	quinine salt (dihydrochloride or sulfate): 10 mg/kg three times a day for 7 days
Option 4	artesunate: 4 mg/kg in a divided loading dose on day 1, followed by 2 mg/kg daily for 6 days.

---

east Asia and Oceania, and 0.25 mg base/kg per day for 14 days in other areas.

It is not necessary to provide anti-relapse treatment to patients living in endemic areas with unabated transmission. In such situations a relapse cannot be distinguished from reinfection and such patients should be treated with an effective blood schizonticide for each symptomatic recurrence of malaria. Pregnant patients in whom primaquine is contraindicated should not be treated until after delivery.

Anti-relapse treatment is usually not feasible in the acute phase of emergencies, but may be appropriate in the chronic phase. It may also have a role during resettlement and repatriation, as discussed at the end of this chapter. However, adherence to the required 14-day treatment course is likely to prove challenging. Shorter courses of anti-relapse treatment, such as the 5-day course adopted in many Asian countries, are ineffective and are not recommended.

Primaquine may be given concurrently with an active blood schizonticide such as chloroquine from the first day of treatment. Primaquine should not be given to a patient who is pregnant or has glucose-6-phosphate dehydrogenase (G6PD) deficiency (the incidence of G6PD deficiency is high in Asia and some parts of Africa), because of the risk of intravascular haemolysis. The patient should be tested for G6PD deficiency before treatment with primaquine: kits that are relatively inexpensive and simple to use are available for this purpose. About 10% of Africans develop a mild, self-limiting haemolysis with a dosage of 15 mg primaquine base per day for 14 days. Severe, life-threatening haemolysis may occur in persons of Asian or Mediterranean origin with a rarer form of G6PD deficiency.

Management of mixed *Plasmodium* infections

Mixed malaria infections with both *P. falciparum* and *P. vivax* occur commonly in many areas of the world, such as Latin America, Ethiopia, Timor-Leste and other parts of north-east Africa and Asia. In these areas, when malaria is diagnosed on clinical grounds, both *P. falciparum* and *P. vivax* infection should be treated. During the acute phase of an emergency, detection of life-threatening *P. falciparum* infection is the main priority, and use of an ACT (except artesunate–SP) will effectively treat both *P. falciparum* and *P. vivax*. If patient numbers are not excessive, microscopy is preferable to RDTs for diagnosis, since it provides reliable species differentiation.

Management of anaemia

Chronic anaemia is common in areas of high malaria transmission and is a particular problem in young children and pregnant women.

Assessment of anaemia (all ages)

- Check for palmar and conjunctival pallor. Time constraints are likely to necessitate oral treatment being started on the basis of clinical signs alone.
- Measure blood haemoglobin (Hb) level. In remote settings, the Haemoglobin Colour Scale (HCS)[1] can be used to check Hb level. Patients with Hb of 10 g/dl or below require oral treatment (see below). Those with Hb <5 g/dl (equivalent to an HCS reading of 6 g/dl or below) *who are symptomatic* (prostration or respiratory distress) (see Box 5.2) must be urgently referred to an inpatient facility for further assessment and possible blood transfusion. Patients with Hb <5 g/dl who are otherwise well can be treated orally.

Treatment of anaemia
Children

- Give ferrous sulfate (200-mg tablet, equivalent to 60 mg elemental iron) once daily for 2 months: 2–12 months $^1/_4$ tablet; 1–5 years $^1/_2$ tablet; >5 years 1 tablet.
- In areas of moderate and high malaria transmission, treat all cases of anaemia in children under 5 years of age with an effective antimalarial drug.
- Treat all children over 2 years of age presumptively for intestinal worms with a single 500-mg dose of mebendazole or 400-mg dose of albendazole (unless either of these has been given in the previous 6 months).
- Advise caregivers about good feeding practices.

---

[1] http://www.who.int/medical_devices/publications/en/HbCS_brochure.pdf,
http://www.who.int/medical_devices/initiatives/anaemia_control/en/

Non-pregnant adults

- Give ferrous sulfate (200-mg tablet, equivalent to 60 mg elemental iron): 1 tablet 3 times a day for 2 months.
- Treat presumptively for intestinal worms with a single 500-mg dose of mebendazole or 400-mg dose of albendazole. The diagnosis should be confirmed by microscopy, if time and facilities allow.

Pregnant women

See "Malaria in special groups", page 97.

Severe falciparum malaria

Management of severe P. falciparum *malaria*

Resuscitation

In complex emergency situations, where patient numbers are high and there are many late presentations, effective triage is essential to identify and treat immediately patients who are at highest risk of dying (see Box 5.2). All patients with signs of severe malaria (see Box 5.3) must receive immediate treatment (see Table 5.1 and Box 5.8). *Prompt resuscitation of patients with severe malaria saves lives.*

Laboratory support

Laboratory support for the management of severe malaria must, at a minimum, include the following:

— accurate microscopy (for the detection of malaria parasites and for examination of cerebrospinal fluid); RDTs can be used as an alternative to malaria microscopy;
— measurement of blood glucose;
— measurement of Hb or packed cell volume (PCV);
— blood grouping and cross-matching, and the ability to screen blood for HIV and hepatitis B.

Nursing care

Regular observation of the patient with severe malaria is critical, because the clinical situation changes quickly. The most important observations are pulse, respiratory rate and pattern, blood pressure, temperature, and level of consciousness. If there is any deterioration in consciousness, it is essential to check for hypoglycaemia and for a significant fall in haemoglobin, because these are amenable to treatment.

Box 5.8 **Supportive and ancillary treatment for patients with severe malaria**

- Clear the airway and check that the patient is breathing.
- Establish intravenous (IV) access.
- Treat convulsions lasting 5 minutes or more (see below).
- Take blood for malaria parasites, blood glucose and haemoglobin. Urea and electrolytes, blood gas and blood culture are also extremely useful, but are unlikely to be feasible in most complex emergency situations.
- Treat hypoglycaemia (blood glucose <2.2 mmol/l) (see below).
- Rapidly assess circulation, hydration and nutritional status, and resuscitate as necessary with normal (0.9%) saline (see below).
- If haemoglobin is <5 g/dl and patient has respiratory distress, transfuse blood.
- For unconscious patients, insert a nasogastric tube and aspirate stomach contents to prevent aspiration pneumonia. Place the patient in the recovery position, and perform a lumbar puncture to exclude meningitis.
- Start antimalarial drug treatment (see below).
- Start antibiotic therapy (see below).

In all patients with severe malaria:

- Check Hb and parasitaemia daily for the first 3 days.

If the patient is unconscious:

- Check blood glucose every 4 hours.
- Check blood glucose and Hb if the level of consciousness deteriorates.

Antimalarial drug treatment

The two options for drug treatment of severe falciparum malaria are the artemisinin derivatives and quinine dihydrochloride (see Box 5.9). Artesunate is the treatment of choice for adults with severe malaria, in view of a recent multi-centre trial in which mortality in the artesunate group was reduced by 34.7% compared with the quinine group.[1] There are still insufficient data for children, however, particularly from high-transmission settings, to permit the same conclusion. An individual patient data meta-analysis of trials comparing artemether and quinine showed no difference in mortality in African children. For children both options are effective if

---

[1] South East Asian Quinine Artesunate Malaria Trial (SEAQUAMAT) group. Artesunate versus quinine for treatment of severe falciparum malaria: a randomised trial. *Lancet*, 2005, 366:717–725.

administered correctly, and the choice between them depends largely on practical considerations.

Intravenous (IV) quinine should be administered by means of a rate-controlled infusion over a period of 4 hours. Because of the risk of fatal hypotension, it should never be given as a bolus IV injection. Intramuscular (IM) quinine can be used for emergency treatment but is associated with the risk of sterile abscess and sciatic nerve palsy. In a complex emergency, it may therefore be more practical to use IM artemether, which is given once daily, has minimal side-effects and clears malaria parasites rapidly.

For the emergency treatment of severe malaria, or of a patient who cannot tolerate oral medication, artesunate can be administered rectally before transport to an inpatient facility. Once the patient is able to tolerate oral medication, treatment must be completed with a full course of an effective oral antimalarial drug – severe malaria will not be cured by a single dose of artesunate (see Box 5.9).

Management of the complications of severe malaria

Management of hypoglycaemia, convulsions, shock, severe anaemia, coma, renal failure, and pulmonary oedema are outlined below:

Treatment of hypoglycaemia (blood glucose <2.2 mmol/l)

- If the patient is able to tolerate oral fluids, give breast milk or a sugar solution (4 level teaspoons (20 grams) of sugar in a 200-ml cup of clean water).

- For unconscious patients or those unable to tolerate oral fluids:
  — Insert an IV line:
    Children: Dilute 50% glucose, 1 ml/kg, in an equal volume of any infusion fluid and give by slow IV injection over a period of 5 minutes. (_Example:_ a child weighing 16 kg would receive 16 x 1 ml = 16 ml 50% glucose diluted to 32 ml). Then follow with a continuous infusion of 5% or (ideally) 10% dextrose.
    Adults: Infuse 50 ml of 50% glucose over 15 minutes.
  — Recheck blood glucose 15 minutes after the end of the infusion.
  — If blood glucose is still <2.2 mmol/l, repeat glucose infusion as above.
  — If it is not possible to insert an IV line and the patient is unconscious, give 1 ml/kg 50% dextrose via nasogastric tube.

- Give oral fluids (breast milk or sugar solution) and food once the patient regains consciousness.

Box 5.9 **Antimalarial drug treatment of severe malaria**

OPTION 1: ARTEMISININ DERIVATIVES
■ **Artemether IM**
Loading dose: 3.2 mg/kg
— Give IM artemether as a single dose on day 1.
  Note: IM artemether should not be given to patients in shock, since absorption is unreliable.
Maintenance dose: 1.6 mg/kg
— Give once a day starting on day 2.
— Continue until the patient is able to tolerate oral medication.
— Treatment should be completed with oral artesunate, 2 mg/kg daily to complete 7 days of treatment, *or* with a single dose of oral SP (in situations where the efficacy of SP is known to be high) or mefloquine, *or* with 3 days of Coartem®.

■ **Artesunate IV or IM**
Loading dose: 2.4 mg/kg
— Give IV over 3 minutes as a single dose on day 1 at 0, 12 and 24 hours.
Maintenance dose: 2.4 mg/kg once daily
— Give IV over 3 minutes once a day beginning on day 2.
— Continue the maintenance dose until the patient is able to tolerate oral medication.
— Treatment should be completed with oral artesunate, 2 mg/kg daily to complete 7 days of treatment, *or* with a single dose of oral SP (in situations where the efficacy of SP is known to be high) or mefloquine (except following a coma or convulsions), *or* with 3 days of Coartem®.

■ **Rectal artesunate**
— Artesunate suppositories should be reserved for situations in which it is not possible to give IV or IM therapy.
— Give 10 mg/kg of artesunate by suppository, and repeat the dose if the suppository is expelled within 1 hour.
— Repeat the dose after 24 hours if it is not possible to refer the patient.
  Note: Artesunate suppositories remain stable in temperatures of up to 40 °C and therefore require cool – but not cold – transport and storage.

OPTION 2: QUININE DIHYDROCHLORIDE
■ **IV administration**
Loading dose: 20 mg salt/kg
— Omit the loading dose if the patient has had an adequate dose of quinine (>40 mg salt/kg) in the previous 2 days. Recent treatment with mefloquine is not a contraindication to a loading dose of quinine.
— The loading dose should be given as an IV infusion over 4 hours (see below).
Maintenance dose: 10 mg salt/kg
— The maintenance dose must be given every 8 hours.

Box 5.9 *Continued*

— The maintenance dose should be given as an infusion over 4 hours (see below).
— If IV therapy is still required after 48 hours, the maintenance dose should be reduced to 7 mg salt/kg to avoid the risk of accumulation.
— A minimum of 3 doses of IV quinine should be given before changing to oral treatment (see below).

Volume of infusion

— Quinine can be diluted in 5% dextrose, 10% dextrose, 4% dextrose–0.18% saline, or normal (0.9%) saline.
— Dilute quinine to a total volume of 10 ml/kg (the same volume is used for both loading and maintenance doses) and infuse over 4 hours.
— To avoid overloading the patient with IV fluids, the volume of the quinine infusion *must* be taken into account when calculating the total 24-hour fluid requirement.
  Example:
  The 24-hour fluid requirement for an adult weighing 50 kg is 50 ml/kg, i.e. 50 x 50 = 2500 ml. The patient will receive 3 x 500-ml infusions of quinine each day = 1500 ml. Therefore, the patient needs an additional 1000 ml of maintenance fluid to bring the 24-hour total to 2500 ml.
— IV quinine can cause hypoglycaemia, and blood glucose should therefore be monitored every 4 hours.

■ **IM administration**

— IM quinine may cause sterile abscesses and should be given only when IV therapy is not possible.
— Dilute quinine 1 part in 5 with normal (0.9%) saline.
— Divide the dose into 2 separate injections and administer by deep IM injection into both anterior thighs (IM quinine should *not* be injected into the buttock).
— A minimum of 3 doses of quinine should be given before changing to oral treatment (see below).

■ **Changing to oral treatment (following IV or IM quinine)**

— Once the patient is able to tolerate oral medication, treatment should be completed with (1) SP + 3 days of artesunate, (2) full course Coartem® (3 days) *or* (3) oral quinine 10 mg salt/kg every 8 hours to complete the remainder of a total of 7 days of quinine treatment. In areas of multidrug-resistant malaria, quinine should be combined with oral clindamycin, 5 mg/kg 3 times a day for 7 days. If clindamycin is unavailable, use oral doxycycline, 3 mg/kg once a day for 7 days, or oral tetracycline, 4 mg/kg 4 times a day for 7 days.
— Doxycycline and tetracycline should *not* be given to children under 8 years or to pregnant women. Clindamycin, however, can safely be given to these groups.
— Mefloquine should be avoided in patients recovering from coma as it increases the risk of post-malaria neurological syndrome.

- If hypoglycaemia is suspected clinically in an unconscious person, and it is not possible to check the blood glucose, give a presumptive infusion of 50% glucose as described above.

  Note: There is a marked risk of hypoglycaemia during the use of quinine in pregnant women and young children.

Treatment of convulsions

- Maintain the airway.

- Turn the patient on his or her side to reduce the risk of aspiration.

- Do not attempt to force anything into the patient's mouth.

- Check blood glucose and treat if <2.2 mmol/l (see above).

- Treat with:
  — diazepam, 0.3 mg/kg (up to a maximum 10 mg), as a slow IV injection over 2 minutes; *or*
  — diazepam, 0.5 mg/kg per rectum, administered by inserting a 1-ml syringe (without a needle) into the rectum; *or*
  — paraldehyde, 0.2 ml/kg (up to a maximum of 10 ml) by deep IM injection into the anterior thigh; *or*
  — paraldehyde, 0.4 ml/kg per rectum.

- If the patient continues to convulse, give further doses of diazepam or paraldehyde every 10 minutes (up to a *maximum of 3 doses* of either drug).

- Treat patients who have multiple (3 or more) or prolonged (lasting 30 minutes or more) convulsions with a loading dose of IM phenobarbital, 10–15 mg/kg.

Fluids

Maintenance fluid requirements (IV, oral, or via nasogastric tube)
Use IV fluids, such as 4% dextrose–0.18% saline or 5% dextrose (ideally with added sodium chloride, 2 mmol/kg per day). Change to 10% dextrose if the patient becomes hypoglycaemic. The following daily maintenance fluid volumes are recommended:

Weight	Daily fluid requirement[a]
<5 kg	150 ml/kg
5–10 kg	120 ml/kg
11–19 kg	80 ml/kg
20–30 kg	60 ml/kg
Child >30 kg and adults	50 ml/kg

[a] The fluid requirement is given in ml per kg body weight per day. The total daily fluid requirement for a 14-kg child would therefore be 14 x 80 = 1120ml, while that for an adult weighing 55 kg would be 55 x 50 = 2750ml.

In most complex emergencies there are large numbers of patients and limited numbers of nursing staff. Close observation of patients is usually impossible, and it is therefore safest to give maintenance fluids by NG tube, in preference to IV infusion. The mother or carer can help to administer NG feeds, which also makes it possible to provide calories in addition to fluid – an important advantage as many patients are likely to be malnourished. The daily fluid requirement can be given as 4-hourly NG feeds (milk or diluted porridge). Inhalation pneumonia must be prevented.

Example:
The daily fluid requirement for a 14-kg child is 80 x 14 ml = 1120ml. This can be given in the form of six 4-hourly NG milk feeds of 187 ml.

Rapid administration of IV fluids for resuscitation of patients in shock or with severe dehydration

- Use normal (0.9%) saline. Note that dextrose solutions, e.g. 5% dextrose, 4% dextrose–0.18% saline, and 10% dextrose, must not be used for fluid resuscitation, since this can lead to cerebral oedema (brain swelling).

- Check that the patient does not have severe malnutrition (severe wasting with associated oedema): patients with severe malnutrition should not be given large volumes of intravenous fluids.

- Children: Infuse 20 ml/kg of normal saline over 15 minutes.

Example:
A child weighing 15 kg would receive 15 x 20 ml = 300 ml.

- Adults: Infuse 1000 ml of normal saline over 30 minutes.

- Reassess the patient. If there is no improvement in hydration or circulation (i.e. pulse becomes slower, capillary refill improves – see Box 5.2), give a second infusion (children: 20 ml/kg normal saline; adults: 1000 ml normal saline).

- Reassess the patient. If there is no improvement in hydration or circulation, give a third infusion (children: 20 ml/kg normal saline; adults: 1000 ml normal saline).

- Reassess the patient. If there is still no improvement in circulation or hydration, infuse 20 ml/kg of blood over 60 minutes.

- Give presumptive treatment with IV antibiotics (see below) to all patients who are in shock, since shock may be secondary to bacteraemia.

Blood transfusion for severe anaemia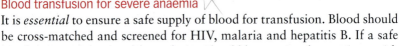

It is *essential* to ensure a safe supply of blood for transfusion. Blood should be cross-matched and screened for HIV, malaria and hepatitis B. If a safe supply cannot be assured, transfusion should be restricted to patients with severe anaemia and signs of acute failure (shock, respiratory distress). If suitable donors without malaria infection cannot be found, blood should be administered with antimalarial treatment.

Children

- Children with Hb <5 g/dl (PCV <15%) and respiratory distress
  - These patients need blood as an *emergency.*
  - Give 20 ml/kg, as packed red cells or whole blood.
  - Infuse the first 10 ml/kg over 30 minutes and the next 10 ml/kg over 2 hours.
  - Reassess the patient at the end of the transfusion. If he or she still has respiratory distress and Hb <5 g/dl, repeat the transfusion.
- Children with Hb <5 g/dl (PCV <15%) but *without* respiratory distress
  - These patients should be transfused but, because their condition is less critical, can be given 20 ml/kg over 3–4 hours.
  - Diuretics (furosemide) are unnecessary.
- Severely malnourished children (severe wasting plus oedema)
  - Give blood much more cautiously to these patients.
  - Infuse 10 ml/kg blood over 3 hours.
  - Give furosemide, 1 mg/kg IV, halfway through the transfusion.

Adults

- Non-pregnant adults
  - Blood transfusion is indicated in patients with Hb <7 g/dl plus symptoms (severe lethargy, prostration, breathlessness). Patients with Hb <7 g/dl who are otherwise asymptomatic and ambulant should not be transfused.

— Blood (500 ml) should be transfused over 3–4 hours.

- Pregnant women
  Blood transfusion is indicated in the following situations:
  — Women of ≥36 weeks gestation with Hb <7 g/dl, even if asymp-
    tomatic (women who are severely anaemic during labour are at
    increased risk of dying).
  — Women of <36 weeks gestation with Hb <7 g/dl plus symptoms
    (severe lethargy, prostration, breathlessness).
  — Transfuse 500 ml blood (packed red cells ideally) slowly over 4–6
    hours. Furosemide, 40 mg IV, should be given halfway through the
    transfusion.
  — Transfusion should be avoided in the third stage of labour because
    of the risk of fluid overload (pulmonary oedema) associated with
    placental separation.

Assessment of level of consciousness

Children aged 5 years and below

The Blantyre coma scale[1] is a means of rapidly assessing and monitoring the
level of consciousness in children. A score of 5 indicates full consciousness,
while a score of 3 or less indicates coma. Ideally, the assessment should be
carried out 4-hourly in all unconscious children.

Response		Score
Motor	Localizes pain[a]	2
	Withdraws in response to pain[b]	1
	No motor response	0
Verbal	Appropriate cry	2
	Inappropriate cry	1
	No cry	0
Eyes	Gaze oriented	1
	Gaze not oriented	0
Total		Maximum 5 (fully conscious)
		Minimum 0 (deep coma)

[a] Apply sternal pressure (the examiner should press firmly on the child's sternum using the knuckles of one hand). A child who is able to localize pain makes an attempt to remove the examiner's hand.

[b] Pressure applied with pencil to nail bed.

[1] Molyneux M et al. Clinical features and prognostic indicators in paediatric cerebral malaria: a study of 131 comatose Malawian children. *Quarterly Journal of Medicine*, 1989, 71(265):441–459.

Children over 5 years of age and adults
Consciousness level should be assessed using the Glasgow coma scale:

Response		Score
Eyes open:	Spontaneously	4
	To speech	3
	To pain	2
	Never	1
Best verbal response:	Oriented	5
	Confused	4
	Inappropriate words	3
	Incomprehensible sounds	2
	None	1
Best motor response:	Obeys commands	5
	Localizes pain[a]	4
	Flexion to pain	3
	Extension to pain	2
	None	1
Total		Minimum 3; Maximum 14[b]

[a] Apply sternal pressure (the examiner should press firmly on the patient's sternum using the knuckles of one hand). A patient who is able to localize pain makes an attempt to remove the examiner's hand.

[b] Unrousable coma is defined as a score of <10.

Ideally, the assessment should be carried out 4-hourly in all unconscious patients, to monitor the level of consciousness.

Management of the unconscious patient

- Ensure that the airway is clear.

- Insert a nasogastric tube and aspirate the stomach contents into a syringe every 4 hours, to reduce the risk of aspiration pneumonia.

- Check that the patient is not hypoglycaemic, shocked, dehydrated, acidotic (breathing pattern) or severely anaemic, and treat any of these conditions urgently (as above).

- Start treatment with artemether, quinine or artesunate (see Box 5.9)

- Perform a lumbar puncture on all unconscious patients to exclude bacterial meningitis. If there is evidence of CSF infection (see Table 5.1) or lumbar puncture is not possible, treat presumptively for bacterial meningitis (see below).

- After successful correction of dehydration and shock, restrict IV fluids to 70% of normal maintenance fluid requirements (described above). Assess fluid balance daily if possible (daily weight gives a rough indication of overall fluid balance).

- Check blood glucose every 4 hours, and Hb and parasitaemia at least daily.

- Treat convulsions that last for >5 minutes (see above).

- Monitor consciousness level every 4 hours with Blantyre coma scale (children 5 years and younger) or Glasgow coma score (children over 5 years of age and adults). If consciousness level deteriorates, check blood glucose and Hb.

- Turn unconscious patients every 4 hours to prevent pressure sores.

Acute renal failure
Children
Established acute renal failure is rare in children with severe malaria, and poor urine output is often secondary to dehydration.

- Patients *must* be catheterized so that urine output can be measured accurately.

- Acute renal failure is suggested by an hourly urine output of <0.5 ml/kg (oliguria).
  Example:
  For a 10-kg child, 0.5ml/kg per hour = 10 x 0.5 = 5 ml/hour. Blood concentrations of urea and creatinine are usually raised.

- Check that oliguria is not due to dehydration or shock by giving test infusion(s) of 20 ml/kg normal (0.9%) saline (see above).

- If, despite correction of dehydration or shock (improved peripheral perfusion, normal blood pressure), hourly urine output is still <0.5 ml/kg, give IV furosemide, 3 mg/kg.

- If urine output remains <0.5 ml/kg per hour, assume that renal failure is established, and restrict fluids to insensible loss (30 ml/kg per day: equivalent to 300 ml/day for a child weighing 10 kg) plus urine output. Consider peritoneal dialysis, if feasible.

Adults

- Patients *must* be catheterized so that urine output can be measured accurately.

- Acute renal failure is suggested by oliguria (urine output <0.4 ml/kg per hour).

- Check that oliguria is not due to dehydration or shock by giving test infusion(s) of 1000 ml normal (0.9%) saline (see above).

- Once dehydration is corrected, give a single dose of furosemide, 40 mg IV. If oliguria persists (<0.4 ml/kg per hour), increase furosemide dose in a stepwise fashion at 60-minute intervals to 100 mg, 200 mg (1-hour infusion), and finally 400 mg (2-hour infusion).

- If urine output remains <0.4 ml/kg per hour, assume that renal failure is established, and restrict fluids to insensible loss (approximately 1000 ml/day) plus urine output. Refer patient to hospital for dialysis if possible. If not, consider peritoneal dialysis, if feasible.

Pulmonary oedema

- Pregnant women are particularly prone to pulmonary oedema, especially during labour and immediately after delivery.

- Check for increased respiratory rate, chest signs (crackles on auscultation) and hepatomegaly.

- If pulmonary oedema is suspected, position the patient upright, give oxygen, stop IV fluids and give IV furosemide, 1 mg/kg.

- If pulmonary oedema is associated with blood transfusion, give IV furosemide, 1 mg/kg, and restart transfusion at a slower rate.

Antibiotics in the management of severe malaria

Patients with severe malaria should be treated with broad-spectrum IV antibiotics in the following circumstances:

- *Severely ill or shocked patients.* A recent study showed that 8% of all children (14% of those <12 months of age) admitted to an African district hospital with severe malaria had concurrent bacteraemia. Mortality was increased 3-fold among those with bacteraemia. All patients who are shocked, or who remain severely ill following resuscitation, should therefore receive presumptive treatment with broad-spectrum IV antibiotics (e.g. ampicillin, 50 mg/kg 6-hourly, plus gentamicin, 7.5mg daily, or according to local patterns of antibiotic resistance).

- *Unconscious patients.* A recent study from an African district hospital showed that 4% of all children (14% of those <12 months of age) with impaired consciousness and malaria parasitaemia had definite evidence of bacterial meningitis. If it is not possible to do a lumbar puncture in an unconscious patient with malaria, or if the CSF findings are suggestive of meningitis, start presumptive IV treatment for meningitis (for example: children – benzylpenicillin, 60 mg/kg 6-hourly, plus chloramphenicol, 25 mg/kg 6-hourly; adults – benzylpenicillin, 5 million IU (600 mg is equivalent to 1 million IU) 6-hourly, plus chloramphenicol, 1000 mg 6-hourly as a standard dose). Treatment should be tailored to local patterns of antibiotic resistance.

All patients with clinical evidence of bacterial infection (e.g. pneumonia, dysentery) should receive antibiotic therapy according to local treatment protocols.

Malaria in special groups
Pregnant women

Plasmodium falciparum is an important cause of maternal and perinatal morbidity and mortality. The clinical effects of falciparum malaria depend to a large extent on the immune status of the woman, which is determined by her previous exposure to malaria, and on her parity.

In pregnant women from areas of low malaria transmission, who have little pre-existing immunity, malaria usually presents as an acute illness, with detectable peripheral parasitaemia. Compared with non-pregnant women, non-immune pregnant women with *P. falciparum* malaria are 2–3 times more likely to develop severe disease and approximately 3 times more likely to die. Women in this group are also at increased risk of miscarriage, stillbirth and neonatal death. Pregnant women often present with life-threatening symptomatic disease, and the clinical course may be complicated by hyperpyrexia (very high fever), hypoglycaemia, severe haemolytic anaemia, pulmonary oedema and cerebral malaria.

Pregnant women living in areas of moderate to high transmission, who have a degree of pre-existing immunity, often develop malaria with few if any symptoms and few if any parasites in the peripheral blood on microscopy, although the placenta may be heavily infected. An RDT may give a positive result, and the woman should be treated. The main maternal effect of malaria infection in these circumstances is anaemia, which is often severe and may be life-threatening when not recognized and treated effectively. The main effect on the baby is low birth weight, a major risk factor for infant death. Pregnant women who are HIV-positive have a higher prevalence and density of malaria parasitaemia than those without HIV infection.

Pregnancy reduces the degree of partial immunity to *P. falciparum* that most women from settings with moderate to high transmission will have acquired during childhood and subsequently; this effect is particularly acute in women in their first and second pregnancies and HIV-positive women during all pregnancies, who are thus at increased risk of malaria infection.

P. vivax infection in pregnancy has less serious consequences than falciparum malaria, and is not associated with severe maternal disease. However, fever can cause miscarriage, stillbirth, and premature delivery. *P. vivax* infection in pregnancy can cause mild maternal anaemia and low birth weight, resulting in increased infant mortality. Pregnant women living in areas with transmission of vivax malaria should therefore be included in prevention and case management strategies.

Options for chemoprophylaxis, intermittent preventive treatment and case management for non-immune and semi-immune pregnant women, as well as management of severe malaria and prevention and management of anaemia in pregnancy are described in the following sections.

Non-immune pregnant women
Chemoprophylaxis
Daily or weekly chemoprophylaxis, which is theoretically an ideal way of preventing malaria in this vulnerable group, is very difficult to achieve in practice. Chloroquine, pyrimethamine and proguanil have been widely used in the past, but adherence to the prophylactic regimens has been poor and resistance to these drugs is now widespread. Weekly prophylaxis with mefloquine was used effectively to prevent both falciparum and vivax malaria in pregnancy in long-term stable refugee camps in south-east Asia, but resistance became widespread by 1998. Mefloquine is no longer a viable option for chemoprophylaxis in parts of this region. In addition, a retrospective study found an increased risk of stillbirth among women treated (as opposed to receiving prophylaxis) with mefloquine compared with other antimalarials.

Screening
The presence of malaria parasites in the peripheral blood of a non-immune adult almost always indicates that he or she has, or will eventually develop, clinical malaria and will require treatment. Consequently, regular screen-

ing and prompt treatment of non-immune pregnant women with parasitae-mia is an effective way of reducing the incidence of severe disease. Weekly screening of women attending antenatal clinics in refugee camps along the Thai–Myanmar border was associated with a significant reduction in ma-ternal and perinatal morbidity and mortality.

In situations where, for security-related or other reasons, antenatal clinic services are not functioning, the provision of an outreach service for the screening of pregnant women (using RDTs or light microscopy for diagnosis) in the community should be considered.

Intermittent preventive treatment

At present, there are no data on the efficacy of intermittent preventive treat-ment (IPT) for preventing the adverse consequences of malaria in pregnant women with no pre-existing immunity to the disease. There is thus no evidence to support the use of IPT in low-transmission areas and during epidemics – in these situations, the focus should be on case management and use of insecticide-treated nets (ITNs).

Semi-immune pregnant women

Asymptomatic malaria infections are common among pregnant women with a partial degree of immunity. A strategy that relies only on passive de-tection and treatment of clinical illness will therefore have little impact on the prevention of anaemia and low birth weight. Interventions for pregnant women in acute complex emergencies in areas of moderate or high *P. fal-ciparum* transmission should be a combination of good case management, active finding of fever cases at community level, proactive screening with microscopy or RDTs of all pregnant women at any point of contact with the health services, priority distribution of ITNs, and provision of IPT as soon as antenatal care (ANC) services have been established.

Intermittent preventive treatment

Intermittent preventive treatment with SP, provided through ANC services, can reduce the incidence of severe anaemia and low birth weight in semi-immune women in areas of moderate to high *P. falciparum* transmission. It is not feasible in acute-phase emergencies unless ANC services already exist.

IPT is an effective, safe and operationally feasible strategy for reducing the burden of malaria among semi-immune pregnant women, even in situ-ations where the health infrastructure is weak. Instead of weekly or daily chemoprophylaxis, IPT involves the administration of a full treatment dose of an effective antimalarial drug, once in the second and once in the third trimester of pregnancy. IPT is given whether or not malaria parasites are detected in the peripheral blood film.

At present, IPT is widely implemented in several African countries (including among refugees and refugee-affected populations in border areas of the United Republic of Tanzania), and is being introduced in many other countries.

A one-dose antimalarial treatment is preferable for IPT, since this enables treatment to be observed at the antenatal clinic and avoids the problems of adherence associated with medication taken at home. Currently, the only drug for which there is documented evidence of effectiveness when used as IPT is SP. In areas where it retains therapeutic efficacy, SP has proved effective in reducing placental parasitaemia, improving birth weight and preventing severe maternal anaemia. Women who are HIV-positive appear to respond less well to IPT with SP than HIV-negative women and should therefore be given IPT on a monthly basis (minimum of 3 doses). Monthly IPT should be given to all pregnant women in situations where the HIV seropositivity rate among women attending antenatal clinics exceeds 10%. IPT with SP should not be given to HIV-positive women who already receive co-trimoxazole prophylaxis. Key points on IPT of semi-immune pregnant women in areas of high malaria endemicity are listed in Box 5.10.

The level of sensitivity required for SP to be effective as IPT is unknown. Therapeutic efficacy of antimalarial drugs is usually measured in children under 5 years of age, and not in semi-immune pregnant women – much less in the context of IPT for semi-immune pregnant women. The following guidance for African countries with intense malaria transmission and ongoing complex emergencies is based on the available evidence:

- *In areas with low or moderate levels of SP resistance* – IPT with SP should be given to all semi-immune pregnant women as soon as ANC services are established, even if no national IPT policy is yet in place.

- *In areas with known relatively high levels of SP resistance* – the situation is less clear. On the one hand, malaria in pregnancy is an important public health problem, and it would be difficult to withhold a prevention strategy that may well still be (partially) effective. On the other hand, it would be difficult to give a (partially) ineffective drug to pregnant women, even if the drug has a good safety profile. Given this dilemma, there is currently insufficient evidence to stop IPT with SP in areas where it is already being used or to introduce it in area where it has not yet been

Box 5.10 **Intermittent preventive treatment of semi-immune pregnant women in areas of high malaria endemicity**

■ Give intermittent preventive treatment with SP (3 tablets) at least twice during pregnancy in women who are HIV-negative, once at the start of the second trimester and once at the start of the third trimester.
■ SP should be given monthly to HIV-positive pregnant women, who are at increased risk of malaria.
■ Monthly IPT should be given to all pregnant women where the HIV seropositivity rate among women attending antenatal clinics exceeds 10%.

Precautions
■ Do *not* give IPT with SP more frequently than once a month. If a woman develops symptomatic disease after receiving SP she should be treated with an alternative antimalarial.
■ Do *not* give SP to women who have a history of allergy to sulfa drugs. If an allergic reaction is suspected after the first IPT dose, do not give further doses.
■ Do *not* give IPT with SP to HIV-positive women who already receive co-trimoxazole prophylaxis.
■ Do *not* give IPT with SP in the first trimester.
■ Advise women to return for the next dose of IPT after a clearly defined time interval, e.g. 3 months.
■ Explain to women that they can still get clinical malaria despite IPT, and that they should return immediately to the clinic if they develop a fever or anaemia.

used. As soon as there is clearer evidence on this issue, it will be available on the WHO web site (www.who.int/malaria/pregnantwomenandinfants.html).

Where IPT programmes are being implemented, IPT should be part of a larger package of prevention and case management strategies targeting pregnant women.

There are insufficient data to allow the use of any other antimalarial regimen to be recommended as an alternative to SP in areas of SP resistance. Further research is needed to establish whether mefloquine is a suitable alternative in areas of SP resistance.

Management of malaria in pregnancy
Non-falciparum malaria
See "Management of non-falciparum malaria" on page 82.

Uncomplicated falciparum malaria

All pregnant women with symptomatic malaria should receive urgent treatment with effective antimalarials. Quinine (and chloroquine and SP where these are still effective) can be used safely for treatment in any trimester, and artesunate, artemether and mefloquine can be used during the second and third trimesters. Artemisinin derivatives should not be withheld in any trimester if they are considered life-saving for the mother. Artemether–lumefantrine is not recommended in the first trimester of pregnancy because of the lack of data. Amodiaquine is apparently safe during pregnancy but only limited published data are available. Primaquine and doxycycline (but not clindamycin) are contraindicated in pregnancy (see Annex IV for more details). It should be noted that the pharmacokinetic properties of most antimalarials are altered in pregnancy and that the recommended dosages could be inadequate, leading to insufficient blood concentrations.

Management of severe malaria in pregnant women

Pregnant women with severe malaria should receive the highest level of inpatient medical care possible because of the high risk of maternal and perinatal mortality. Hypoglycaemia, acute pulmonary oedema, hyperpyrexia, postpartum haemorrhage, premature delivery and perinatal death are particular risks.

Antimalarial drug treatment

Severe malaria in pregnant women should be treated with IV quinine, IM artemether or IV artesunate (see Box 5.9). Intravenous quinine is safe in all three trimesters of pregnancy but may induce hypoglycaemia. When available, IV artesunate is the treatment of choice in the second and third trimesters of pregnancy. The safety of these drugs in the first trimester has not been established, and quinine should therefore be used during early pregnancy. *Neither quinine nor artemisinin derivatives should be withheld in any trimester if they are considered life-saving for the mother.*

Presentation and treatment of complications

- *Hypoglycaemia.* Hypoglycaemia is a significant risk for all pregnant women with malaria. It may occur during the clinical course of uncomplicated malaria, may be asymptomatic, or may present with sweating, confusion, agitated behaviour, drowsiness, convulsions or loss of consciousness. Women in the second and third trimesters of pregnancy who are undergoing treatment with IV quinine are at particularly high risk, and this risk persists for several days postpartum.

102

In patients with cerebral malaria, hypoglycaemia may be asymptomatic or may cause a deterioration in the level of consciousness, extensor posturing, or convulsions. Differential diagnoses include sepsis, meningitis and eclampsia. Hypoglycaemia may also recur after correction with IV glucose.

For these reasons, *regular monitoring (at least 4-hourly) of the blood glucose of all pregnant women with severe malaria is extremely important*, particularly if they are receiving treatment with quinine. Blood glucose must be checked if there is any change in the level of consciousness, and immediate treatment must be given if it is <2.2 mmol/l. See "Treatment of hypoglycaemia", page 87.

- *Acute pulmonary oedema.* Acute pulmonary oedema commonly develops immediately after delivery, but may occur at any time during the first week postpartum. Severe anaemia and the increase in blood volume and peripheral resistance that follows placental separation may precipitate acute pulmonary oedema and heart failure. This is a medical emergency that requires immediate treatment.
  - Pregnant women are particularly prone to pulmonary oedema, especially during labour and immediately after delivery.
  - Check for increased respiratory rate, chest signs (crackles on auscultation), and hepatomegaly.
  - If pulmonary oedema is suspected, position the patient upright, give oxygen, stop IV fluids, and give IV furosemide, 1 mg/kg.
  - If pulmonary oedema is associated with blood transfusion, give furosemide, 1 mg/kg IV, and restart transfusion at a slower rate.

- *Severe anaemia.* Blood transfusion is indicated in the following situations:
  - Women of ≥36 weeks gestation with Hb <7 g/dl, PCV <21% (even if asymptomatic – women who are severely anaemic during labour are at increased risk of dying).
  - Women of <36 weeks gestation with Hb <7 g/dl plus symptoms (severe lethargy, prostration, breathlessness).
  - Women of <36 weeks gestation with Hb <5 g/dl (PCV <15%).

Transfuse 500 ml blood (packed red cells ideally) slowly over 4–6 hours. Furosemide, 40 mg IV, should be given halfway through the transfusion. Transfusion should be avoided in the third stage of labour because of the risk of fluid overload (pulmonary oedema) associated with placental separation.

It is essential to ensure that the blood supply is "safe". Local laboratory facilities must therefore be able to perform compatibility testing (cross-matching) and screening for HIV, malaria and, if possible, hepatitis B. If suitable donors without malaria infection cannot be found, the blood should be administered with an antimalarial treatment.

Prevention and treatment of anaemia in pregnant women

Anaemia is a common, and potentially dangerous, complication of pregnancy. The prevention of anaemia should, therefore, be a priority for all health programmes dealing with pregnant women.

- Ferrous sulfate, 200 mg (equivalent to 60 mg elemental iron), plus folic acid, 0.25 mg, should be given daily throughout pregnancy.

- In areas of moderate and high malaria transmission, where there is a high risk of asymptomatic malaria infection in pregnancy, pregnant women should be given IPT with SP, once in the second and once in the third trimester.

- Pregnant women who are anaemic (Hb 10 g/dl or below) should be given ferrous sulfate, 200 mg (equivalent to 60 mg elemental iron) 3 times daily, and folic acid, 0.25 mg 3 times daily, for 2 months.

- Presumptive treatment for intestinal worms (using a single 500-mg dose of mebendazole or 400-mg dose of albendazole) can be given once in the second or third trimester of pregnancy. Note that these drugs should not be given in the first trimester. The diagnosis should be confirmed by microscopy, if time and facilities allow.

Malnourished persons
Management of uncomplicated malaria

Malnutrition is a significant cause of mortality and morbidity in complex emergencies, and is associated with an increased risk of a poor outcome from severe malaria.

Diagnosis

Patients with severe malnutrition (<70% of median weight-for-height, or <–3SD[1]) may have asymptomatic malaria infection and should therefore be

---

[1] SD = standard deviation score or Z-score. A weight-for-height of –2SD indicates the child is at the lower end of the normal range, and <–3SD indicates severe wasting. A weight-for-height of –3SD is approximately equivalent to 70% of the weight-for-height of the average (median) child (source and reference values: http://www.who.int/child-adolescent-health/publications/referral_care/chap7/chap7fr.htm).

Box 5.11 **Therapeutic feeding in the Republic of the Congo**

MSF France established therapeutic feeding centres to treat severely malnourished children returning from the Republic of the Congo in May 1999. There were large numbers of malnourished children with severe malaria and a shortage of qualified staff. Standard management with IV quinine infusion 3 times a day was operationally difficult and potentially dangerous, so the following protocol was introduced:

- Clinical diagnosis of malaria was confirmed by RDT (Paracheck®, 98% positive, $n = 231$).
- Combination therapy with IM artemether once a day for 3 days combined with a single dose of sulfadoxine–pyrimethamine on day 3.

High rates of clinical recovery were achieved. Artemether was easy to use, and no side-effects were noted.

screened for malaria – using microscopy or RDT – on admission to a therapeutic feeding centre and weekly thereafter until discharge. Once a patient has tested positive for malaria, further weekly screening can be done only with microscopy.

Treatment

The absorption and bioavailability of several antimalarial drugs, including chloroquine and quinine, can be significantly impaired in patients with severe malnutrition. Increasing antimalarial drug bioavailability may reduce the risk of treatment failure due to poor drug absorption. All oral antimalarial drugs should be administered together with food, as this helps to increase absorption.

Treatment failures should be treated with either the 7 days of IM artemether, or with IV quinine (see Box 5.9). Intramuscular artemether is the preferred option for ease of administration, rapid parasite clearance and minimal adverse side-effects, but it should not be given to patients in vascular shock.

Management of severe malaria

Patients with severe malaria and severe malnutrition are at very high risk of death and require intensive medical and nursing care. They should be hospitalized in a therapeutic feeding centre and treated with an effective IM or IV antimalarial regimen (see Boxes 5.9 and 5.11), preferably using an artemisinin derivative.

Returning refugees and internally displaced populations

In general, mass population movements in geographical areas of mixed endemicity may result in the arrival of large numbers of people with malaria parasites in areas where there is normally little transmission, and the arrival of non-immune populations in areas where there is moderate or intense transmission. It is also possible that people will bring with them different parasite species (notably falciparum), or strains of malaria parasites that are more resistant to certain antimalarial drugs than the local strains. These situations pose a health risk for the resident populations and/or for the new arrivals.

The incidence of *P. falciparum* malaria relative to that of *P. vivax* has, for example, increased in the border region between Afghanistan and Tajikistan during the past decade, partly as a result of the cross-border movements of Afghan refugees.

If there is a risk that organized repatriation of displaced populations could introduce or re-introduce malaria or drug-resistant malaria, preventive measures should be considered. The most cost-effective measure is mass screening and selective treatment of individuals with malaria, which should be carried out as close as possible to the time of departure and entails the following:

— screening the entire returning population with a diagnostic test;
— treating individuals with malaria with effective antimalarial drugs that have blood schizonticidal and gametocytocidal activity, such as ACT.

In areas where *P. vivax* and *P. ovale* are prevalent, treatment would need to include anti-relapse treatment with primaquine. However, primaquine treatment should be given only to individuals who test negative for G6PD, and needs to be continued for 14 days. This may not be operationally feasible with large population groups.

Because of the incubation period of malaria, some individuals may develop parasitaemia and symptoms only once they are back home. Returnees should thus receive health education messages regarding malaria symptoms and the need to seek treatment if they fall ill with fever back home. Local clinics that may be unaccustomed to seeing malaria patients must be instructed about timely and adequate diagnosis and treatment of these patients.

Partial immunity will decrease during stays of 6 months or more in non-endemic areas. When refuges are repatriated after a long stay in an

Box 5.12 **Malaria management in complex emergencies –**
summary of key points

Good triage, diagnosis and case management are among the most
effective ways of reducing avoidable illness and death from malaria.

Triage
- Emergency triage is essential. The priority should be to save lives,
and the sickest patients need to be treated first. The key is the rapid
identification, assessment and treatment of emergency danger signs.

Diagnosis
- Differential clinical assessment and laboratory confirmation of
diagnosis are essential aspects of malaria case management in complex
emergencies. Clinical assessment alone is very inaccurate, as the clinical
presentation of malaria (both uncomplicated and severe) is variable and
nonspecific. Patients often have more than one underlying disease, and all
conditions must be rapidly identified and appropriately treated.
- Rapid diagnostic tests and microscopy are the two tools used for the
diagnosis of malaria.
- In acute emergencies, limited time and resources make rapid diagnostic
tests preferable to microscopy for screening populations, for confirmation
of clinical diagnosis in low-transmission areas, and for confirming malaria
in severely ill patients in moderate- to high-transmission areas.

Case management
- Factors determining the choice of antimalarial drugs include drug
efficacy and resistance, patient case-load, access and adherence, drug
availability, and ease of administration.
- Uncomplicated *P. falciparum* malaria in acute emergencies should be
treated with artemisinin-based combination therapy (ACT).
- Uncomplicated non-falciparum malaria is normally treated with
chloroquine. In areas of chloroquine resistance, mefloquine, quinine and
artesunate are effective alternatives.
- In areas where *P. falciparum* and *P. vivax* are common, patients should
be treated for both species, if microscopy is not possible.
- Severe malaria should be treated with artemisinin derivatives or
quinine. For children, both options are effective if administered correctly;
IM artemether is easier to administer. Artesunate is the treatment of
choice for adults with severe malaria.
- To reduce mortality, close monitoring and immediate treatment of
complications of severe malaria are essential.

Continued page 108

Box 5.12 *Continued*

Priority vulnerable groups for active detection of fever cases and screening
■ Pregnant women, children under 2 years of age, severely malnourished children (therapeutic feeding centres).
■ Children under 5, and people known to be HIV-positive or with strong clinical suspicions of AIDS.
■ Affected population in general, especially (newly) non-immune people arriving in endemic area.

area with little or no transmission to an area with higher transmission, the entire population will be at risk of severe malaria disease and death.

When organized repatriation of displaced populations could re-expose previously semi-immune populations (*who have now lost their immunity*) to malaria transmission, an intense IEC (information, education and communication) campaign on the new risks of malaria should be organized, and can be accompanied by distribution of ITNs. The focus should be on personal protection methods (strict use of ITNs) and the need for early diagnosis and prompt treatment of all fever episodes. In the receiving area, local health workers may be unaccustomed to the dangers of malaria infection for non-immune older children and adults, and must be instructed about timely and adequate diagnosis and treatment of these patients.

Further reading

WHO (2000). *Bench aids for the diagnosis of malaria*, 2nd ed. Geneva, World Health Organization.

WHO (2000). Severe falciparum malaria. *Transactions of the Royal Society of Tropical Medicine and Hygiene*, 94(1):S1–S90.

WHO (2004). *The use of malaria rapid diagnostic tests*. Manila, World Health Organization Regional Office for the Western Pacific (available at www.wpro.who.int/rdt/docs/RDTGuidelines_final.pdf

WHO (2005). *Malaria treatment guidelines*. Geneva, World Health Organization (in press).

Finding out more

Malaria in Emergencies Network
Fax: +41 22 791 4824
E-mail: rbmemergencies@who.int

Assistance can also be obtained through:

Dr Peter Bloland
Centers for Disease Control and Prevention
Atlanta, GA
USA
E-mail: Pbb1@cdc.gov

and

Dr François Nosten
Shoklo Malaria Research Unit
736/2 Intrakiri Road
P.O. Box 46
Mae Sod, 63110
Tak, Thailand
E-mail: SMRU@tropmedres.ac

CHAPTER 6

Prevention

This chapter
■ discusses the methods available for malaria prevention
■ outlines how to make decisions about prevention interventions and how to organize prevention activities
■ describes features of the mosquito life cycle relevant to malaria prevention.

Malaria prevention in complex emergencies

While the first priorities in the acute phase of an emergency are prompt and effective diagnosis and treatment of people with malaria, prevention can make an important contribution to reducing the risk of infection and saving lives. Malaria prevention strategies include vector control and personal protection against mosquito bites, in addition to intermittent preventive treatment during pregnancy to avert severe anaemia and low birth weight.

Chapter 4 addresses prevention during malaria outbreaks, and information about prevention in pregnant women is included in Chapter 5. This chapter deals with mosquito vectors, vector control, and personal protection against mosquito bites.

In emergency situations where there is a risk of malaria, the most important initial questions related to prevention are:

- Is malaria prevention likely to be useful? (How great is the malaria burden? Where is transmission occurring?)
- Is malaria prevention feasible? (What is the situation regarding access, security, population mobility, human resources, funding, logistics?)

Assessment of the situation (see Chapter 2) – and particularly finding out about the malaria control strategy in the host country or in the country of origin of the refugee population – should provide some of the answers to these questions. However, the nature of complex emergencies presents both opportunities and constraints (see Box 6.1) that may justify a different approach to prevention.

Box 6.1 **Factors in complex emergencies that may affect the approach to prevention**

Opportunities
- Readily available trained workforce and adequate supervision.
- Concentration of population, which may facilitate access, health education and logistics.
- Additional humanitarian funding provided by international donor organizations.

Constraints
- Access to the population limited by conflict.
- Priority for curative care and feeding the population may limit funds and manpower available for vector control.
- Most malaria transmission may occur outside resettlement sites or camps.
- Language barriers may make it difficult to provide information and education.
- Lack of expertise in vector control.
- Rapid staff turnover.
- Temporary shelters differ from local housing and may make indoor residual spraying and the use of ITNs more problematic.
- Unstable and unpredictable situations make longer-term planning more difficult.
- Evaluation of prevention strategies is more difficult.
- Problems in securing orders and importing commodities (insecticide, pumps, nets) quickly enough.

There are also unanswered questions about malaria prevention in complex emergencies, such as whether vector control is an appropriate response to outbreaks or can be implemented quickly enough to make a difference (see Chapter 8).

The approach to malaria prevention will also change as a complex emergency situation moves from the acute phase to the chronic phase.

- In acute-phase crises the priorities are prompt and effective treatment of all clinical malaria episodes, to limit avoidable malaria deaths. Where feasible, this can be supplemented with barrier methods of mosquito-bite prevention for targeted individuals or priority vulnerable groups at high risk of severe malaria and death. Exceptionally, indoor residual spraying with insecticides – which requires substantial advance planning, logistics and human and material resources – may be possible to protect people in well-organized settings such as transit camps.

- In chronic crises, as the situation stabilizes, it may be possible to prevent new infections by the addition of high-coverage community vector control measures – covering a high percentage of the population with insecticide-treated materials or spraying a high percentage of dwellings with residual insecticide to achieve an impact on transmission.

Acute phase

During the acute phase, decisions about whether or not to implement malaria prevention and about the choice of prevention methods will depend on:

— the risk of infection;
— the behaviour of the population (e.g. mobility, sleeping arrangements);
— the type of shelter available (e.g. plastic sheeting, tents, permanent housing);
— the behaviour of the local vector.

For example, in situations where the population is on the move, it will not be possible to spray houses but insecticide-treated mosquito nets or materials may be appropriate. Where people have no tradition of net use or shelter is very basic, insecticide-treated materials may be more acceptable and feasible than nets.

Chronic phase

As the situation stabilizes, longer-term approaches can be introduced. Different prevention methods may also be needed as the population becomes less mobile and temporary shelters are replaced by more permanent structures. For example, there may be greater opportunities for providing information and education to the population about personal protection methods.

Prevention methods

Methods that are appropriate for complex emergencies

Indoor residual spraying

Indoor residual spraying (IRS) involves spraying a persistent insecticide onto the inside walls and ceilings or the underside of the roof and eaves of houses, in order to kill mosquitoes when they come indoors to feed and rest. The basic preconditions for IRS are:

— an endophilic malaria vector (i.e. mosquitoes enter and rest inside houses for long enough to absorb the insecticide);

— an insecticide to which the vector is susceptible; and
— a population living in dwellings with sprayable surfaces.

To be effective as a community control measure, IRS requires coverage of at least 85% of dwellings, ensuring that the majority of mosquitoes are exposed to the insecticide.

Indoor sleeping is not strictly a requirement for IRS success. In Afghan refugee camps, for example, people sleep outdoors on hot summer nights, but indoor spraying still provides protection against malaria because mosquitoes rest indoors during the day.

Given the operational requirements, IRS is most suited to areas with some stability where advance planning and close monitoring of campaign coverage are possible. In acute-phase emergencies, there may be opportunities for IRS during advance planning for refugee transit camps and other well-organized settings.

An IRS campaign requires substantial advance planning, logistic support, and human and material resources. Its effectiveness is highly dependent on operational factors – timely delivery of commodities, on-site expertise and capacity, trained staff, good organization and planning, manpower, supervision, and appropriate IEC (information, education, communication). Timing is critical – at least 85% of the walls, ceilings, etc. must be sprayed with insecticide before the expected peak transmission season.

Good-quality compression sprayers that comply with WHO specifications must be used for IRS: mechanical pumps are prone to wear and tear. These may need to be imported, together with spare parts and the insecticide, and this takes time and requires adequate planning. Proper maintenance is important to ensure that compression sprayers are efficient and that their working life is maximized: IRS campaigns have been known to fail because of neglect of spray pump maintenance. The insecticide must be applied safely, and the operations must be properly supervised. Spray teams require at least 2 days' intensive theoretical and practical training before they can start field operations, which must then be closely supervised and monitored. In view of these various requirements, IRS campaigns are not always carried out well even when the required operational factors are all in place.

WHO has produced an illustrated manual that can be used for training spray teams – *Manual for indoor residual spraying: application of residual sprays for vector control* (WHO, 2000). This manual is intended to serve as a model for the development of relevant training materials and procedures at country level.

Important aspects of interactions between spray teams and target households are summarized in Box 6.2.

Table 6.1 lists the insecticides commonly used for residual spraying, recommended application rates (g/m^2), and the residual life or persistence. Any of the insecticides recommended by WHO can be used if available locally and known to be effective. WHO specifications for public health pesticides – for quality control and international trade – are available at www.who.int/whopes/quality.

If malaria transmission is seasonal, it is important to spray just before or at the start of the season. If there is an outbreak, spraying is useful only if the insecticide is on the walls before the peak of the epidemic is reached. This requires detailed advance planning and considerable logistic capacity and is rarely possible in practice. Delayed IRS is a waste of resources as it may have little impact on malaria transmission or on a malaria outbreak (see Box 6.3).

Box 6.2 **Household aspects of indoor residual spraying**

Household preparations
- Inform the occupants of the household of the spraying schedule and the reasons for spraying.
- Allow the occupants time to prepare and vacate the living areas.
- Remove all household items, including water, food, cooking utensils and toys. Items that cannot be removed should be well covered.
- Move pets and domestic animals away from the house/hut.
- Occupants *must* leave before spraying begins.
- Areas occupied by sick people who cannot be moved must not be sprayed.

Household procedures after spraying
- Advise occupants to stay outside while the spray is drying.
- Instruct occupants to sweep or mop the floor before children and pets are allowed to re-enter.
- Instruct occupants not to clean the sprayed surfaces.

Waste disposal
- Put washings from sprayer into pit latrines or into pits dug for the purpose (away from sources of drinking-water).
- Never pour insecticide into rivers, pools or drinking-water sources.
- Never reuse empty insecticide containers, and do not burn them.

Table 6.1 **WHO-recommended insecticides for indoor residual spraying against malaria vectors[a]**

Insecticide compounds and formulations[b]	Class[c]	Dosage (g/m²)	Mode of action	Duration of effective action (months)
Alpha-cypermethrin, WP & SC	P	0.02–0.03	contact	4–6
Bendiocarb, WP	C	0.1–0.4	contact & airborne	2–6
Bifenthrin, WP	P	0.025–0.050	contact	3–6
Cyfluthrin, WP	P	0.02–0.05	contact	3–6
DDT[d], WP	OC	1–2	contact	>6
Deltamethrin, WP & WG	P	0.020–0.025	contact	3–6
Etofenprox, WP	P	0.1–0.3	contact	3–6
Fenitrothion, WP	OP	2	contact & airborne	3–6
Lambda-cyhalothrin, WP	P	0.02–0.03	contact	3–6
Malathion, WP	OP	2	contact	2–3
Pirimiphos-methyl, WP & EC	OP	1–2	contact & airborne	2–3
Propoxur, WP	C	1–2	contact & airborne	3–6

[a] Source: Najera JA, Zaim M (2003). *Malaria vector control: decision-making criteria and procedures for judicious use of insecticides*. Geneva, World Health Organization (WHO/CDS/WHOPES/2002.5 Rev.1).

[b] EC = emulsifiable concentrate; SC = suspension concentrate; WG = water-dispersible granules; WP = wettable powder.

[c] OC = organochlorine; OP = organophosphate; C = carbamate; P = pyrethroid.

[d] For the conditions for using DDT, see: *Stockholm Convention on Persistent Organic Pollutants (POPs)* (2001), United Nations Environment Programme (UNEP/CHEMICALS/2001/3), page 49.

Effect of the surfaces to be sprayed

The nature of the surface to be sprayed and the insecticide formulation chosen affect both the availability of the insecticide and the duration of its residual effect. Generally, surfaces of organic origin – wood, bamboo, leaves, thatch, etc. – and metals are not absorptive; persistence on these surfaces is therefore related to the volatility of the insecticide (which depends, in turn, on temperature and the characteristics of the formulation). In contrast, insecticide may be absorbed into mud surfaces, the extent of absorption depending on the particle size of the insecticide. Heat from the sun may inactivate insecticide deposits. Alkaline surfaces such as whitewashed walls will inactivate organophosphates, carbamates and pyrethroids.

Box 6.3 **Impact of spraying on malaria incidence (per 100 person-years)[1]**

A. Spraying with malathion in a group of Afghan camps in July 1992 at the start of the transmission season prevented most transmission

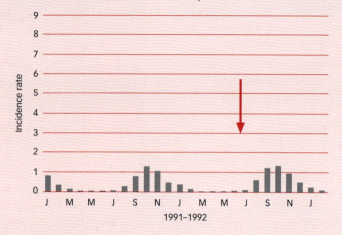

B. Late spraying in a group of neighbouring camps in Sept–Oct 1992 failed to curb the outbreak (which came to a natural end in the winter). This illustrates the importance of correct timing of spray campaigns at the onset of the transmission season

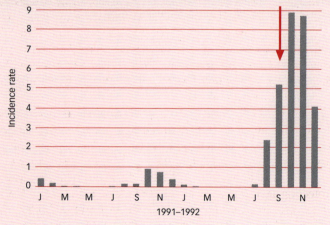

[1] Source: Rowland M (1995). Unpublished report to UNHCR on Afghan refugee malaria control programme. HealthNet International.

Programme monitoring
Monitoring of programme quality should take place during the IRS application (indicators a–d below) and 1 month afterwards (indicator e):

a) Coverage = number of dwellings sprayed/number of dwellings in targeted area (%).
b) Insecticide used per dwelling = quantity of insecticide used/number of dwellings sprayed (a measure of efficiency and correct use of insecticide).
c) User acceptability pre-spray = % of households refusing to be sprayed.
d) % of spray pumps properly maintained and still working during and at the end of the campaign.
e) User acceptability post-spray = % of dwellings replastered or washed, or % of householders complaining about IRS.

Insecticide-treated mosquito nets

Sleeping under an untreated mosquito net provides a physical barrier against mosquitoes – but mosquitoes can still bite if there is a small hole or tear in the net or if any part of the body is touching the net. Treating nets with a suitable insecticide increases the level of protection: the insecticide kills or repels mosquitoes before they can enter the net or bite the person sleeping under the net. Insecticide treatment of nets provides personal protection for all those who sleep under them even when coverage is low. High coverage of the population (≥60%, although some studies indicate 50%) with insecticide-treated nets (ITNs) can reduce the adult mosquito population and may therefore also protect people who do not use ITNs. In Africa, ITNs work well against all malaria vector species *if used regularly and correctly*. Distribution of untreated nets is not recommended because when they become torn or holed, as they inevitably will, they offer little or no protection against mosquitoes.

In recent years, ITNs have been shown to be very effective in reducing malaria mortality and morbidity in the chronic phase of complex emergencies. For example, even limited distribution of ITNs has reduced malaria mortality and morbidity in Afghan refugee camps: 3 years after receiving free nets, 65% of refugees were still using them and achieving better than 70% protection against malaria attacks (Rowland et al., 1997). The impact in other refugee situations has been mixed; for example ITNs have been effective in Viet Nam (Cong & Schapira, 1998) but less effective in refugee camps on the Thai–Myanmar border (Luxemburger et al., 1996).

Nets vary in size and are made from a variety of fabrics. Long-lasting insecticidal nets are preferable in complex emergencies to avoid the need for treating and drying nets in the field, and for regular re-treatment. If long-lasting nets are not available, insecticide treatment of conventional ITNs in the presence of the recipients is preferable to distribution of pretreated nets, because of problems in ensuring the use of good-quality insecticide products and proper dosing of pretreated nets. Moreover, if the presence of insecticide is not apparent to recipients of pretreated nets, as is often the case, they are less likely to seek re-treatment of their nets later. Finally, experience indicates that organizations that distribute pretreated nets often fail to provide re-treatment 6 months later. In Afghanistan, it was found that dipping the nets in front of the recipients was essential to stimulate appropriate use and later re-treatment.

The easiest method for treating nets on the spot involves simple plastic bags, each large enough to contain a net plus the appropriate volume of water. Treatment consists of adding 500 ml (for a synthetic net) or 2 litres (for a cotton net) of water to a bag, plus a dose of insecticide, mixing thoroughly, introducing the net and making a knot in the bag. Users are then asked to soak the net in the solution contained in the bag and to dry it once they are back home or in their shelters. This method is simple, limits queuing, and takes little time for either users or dippers – although subsequent disposal of bags may be problematic. The quantities of insecticide needed per treated net are listed in Table 6.2.

Table 6.2 **WHO-recommended insecticides for treatment of mosquito nets**[a]

Insecticide	Formulation[b]	Dose[c] for one net (any size)
Deltamethrin	25% WT	1 tablet
	1% SC	40 ml
Lambda-cyhalothrin	2.5% CS	10 ml
Alpha-cypermethrin	10% SC	6 ml
	6% SC	10 ml
Cyfluthrin	5% EW	15 ml
Etofenprox	10% EW	30 ml
Permethrin	10% EC	75 ml

[a] Source: WHO (2000). *Instructions for treatment and use of insecticide-treated mosquito nets.* Geneva, World Health Organization (WHO/CDS/RBM/2002.41, available at www.who.int/malaria/cmc_upload/0/000/016/007/InstructionsITNen1.pdf).

[b] EC = emulsifiable concentrate; SC = suspension concentrate; CS = microencapsulated; EW = oil-in-water emulsion

[c] The dose for one net may be provided as a tablet, small bottle or sachet of liquid, or the insecticide may be supplied in bulk. Mix one dose of insecticide with the recommended amount of water (500 ml for a synthetic net, 2 litres for a cotton net) to treat one net of any size.

Depending on the persistence of the insecticide used, the frequency of net washing, and the seasonality of malaria transmission, ITNs normally need to be re-treated every 6–12 months. The amount of insecticide needed to treat enough nets for a family is less than the amount required to spray the walls and ceiling of a house. Net treatment thus costs less than house spraying – but the cost of providing nets may be higher than the cost of two or three rounds of IRS.

Long-lasting insecticide-treated nets (LLINs) are increasingly available. These are factory-treated mosquito nets that are expected to retain their biological activity for a minimum number of standard WHO washes and a minimum period of time under field conditions. Currently, an LLIN would be expected to retain biological activity for at least 20 standard WHO washes under laboratory conditions and 3 years of recommended use under field conditions.[1] This makes them very attractive for use in emergency situations despite their higher cost compared with conventional nets. The only LLINs currently recommended by WHO for malaria prevention and control are Olyset Net® and PermaNet® 2.0; in December 2003 PermaNet® 2.0 received an interim recommendation requiring further large-scale field studies to confirm long-lasting efficacy for prevention and control of malaria and other vector-borne diseases in different settings. The wash resistance of PermaNet® 2.0 over 20 washes was recently demonstrated in an Afghan refugee camp (Graham et al., 2005). More information is available on the RBM and WHOPES web sites. LLINs made of polyethylene are stronger and more durable (www.who.int/whopes/quality/en/OlysetInterimSpecification.pdf). Institutional buyers should follow the WHO 2001 guidelines *Specifications for netting materials* (available at www.who.int/malaria/cmc_upload/0/000/012/756/ netspex.pdf).

Nets can be used indoors or outdoors. Indoors, they can be suspended from walls or ceilings using string or guy ropes. Outdoors, nets can be supported on poles; rounded poles should be used to avoid damaging the netting and care is needed to hold them firmly in position (Rozendaal, 1997). Before nets are distributed, it is important to find out about sleeping practices and consult the population on how nets can best be suspended or supported. Distribution of nets must be accompanied by information and, if necessary, materials to enable people to use them correctly. Information

---

[1] Source: WHO (2005). *Guidelines for laboratory and field testing of long-lasting insecticidal mosquito nets.* Geneva, World Health Organization (WHO/CDS/WHOPES/GCDPP/2005.11).

and pictorial leaflets about treated nets should also emphasize the importance of not washing nets, of keeping them out of sunlight and rain, and on the need for timely re-treatment.

An illustrated manual – *Instructions for treatment and use of insecticide-treated mosquito nets* – that can be used for training and health education messages is available at www.who.int/malaria/cmc_upload/0/000/016/007/InstructionsITNen1.pdf.

Because of the behavioural change needed to make ITN interventions a success, community distribution of treated nets in acute emergencies is an option only if the target community is already in the habit of using nets. Where community vector control interventions (IRS) are already ongoing, community ITN distribution in acute crises is unnecessary. Distribution of ITNs should initially target high-priority vulnerable groups who are biologically at increased risk of severe disease and who thus benefit most from the personal protection effect, as outlined in Box 6.4.

The quality and likely effectiveness of the intervention should be assessed by monitoring at the time of distribution (to track coverage) and 1 month and 6 months later (to determine appropriate use and retention), using the following indicators:

a) Coverage = number of ITNs distributed/target population size (%).
b) Utilization rate = number of people using ITNs/number of people given ITNs (%).
c) Retention rate = number of people retaining ITNs/number of people originally given ITNs (%).
d) Deterioration rate = average number of holes per ITN.

> *Note:* Even nets with some holes can be protective against mosquitoes if they are treated with pyrethroid insecticide – this is one of the purposes of the insecticide treatment. Knowing the deterioration rate allows further purchases of ITNs to replace grossly damaged nets to be planned.

Methods with limited evidence base, deserving further local research in operational settings

Conventional vector control interventions (ITN, IRS) are in general not feasible for acute-phase emergencies. New vector control tools for acute emergencies are needed that:

— place little or no extra burden on implementing agencies;
— can be stockpiled long term; and
— require little or no behavioural change among implementers and users.

Box 6.4 **ITN distribution by phase of emergency, level of transmission**

Acute-phase emergencies in areas of high/moderate transmission

1. Use ITNs for all beds/patients in hospitals and therapeutic feeding centres (TFC), and provide ITNs to the households of TFC patients on discharge.
2. Distribute ITNs to pregnant women and children under 2 years of age *provided that* the following three preconditions are met:
   — ITNs have been stockpiled in advance
   — the community is used to using them
   — no community vector control interventions (IRS) are ongoing.
3. Finally, *if supplies remain* after situations 1 and 2 have been taken care of:
   — provide ITNs through supplementary feeding centres to the household of every enrolled child on first contact;
   — distribute ITNs to children under 5 years of age (provided that the preconditions listed under 2 above are met);
   — distribute ITNs to the entire households of pregnant women and children under 2 of age (extend to 5 years of age if supplies allow).

Acute-phase emergencies in low-transmission areas of Africa

Use ITNs only in clinical settings (TFC beds, hospital beds); no community distribution schemes.

Chronic-phase emergencies in areas of high/moderate transmission

1. Ensure that ITN distribution for acute-phase emergency is met.
2. Extend ITN coverage to the entire households of pregnant women and children under 2 years of age, with catch-up distribution schemes through antenatal care, immunization programmes and primary health care.
3. Distribute ITNs through regular catch-up distribution schemes to people with known HIV infection or strong clinical suspicion of AIDS.
4. Finally, if supplies remain after 1, 2 and 3 have been completed:
   — extend ITN coverage to entire households of children under 5 years of age with catch-up distribution schemes through immunization programmes and primary health care;
   — extend ITN distribution to the affected population in general.

Chronic-phase emergencies in low-transmission areas of Africa

Interventions as for chronic-phase emergencies in areas of high/moderate transmission.

Insecticide-treated blankets and plastic sheeting are the most promising tools but have not yet passed WHOPES evaluation. These methods – and others that have been shown to be appropriate for complex emergencies in certain settings (mainly Asia) but whose application in other parts of the world would require local operational research – are discussed in the paragraphs that follow.

Other insecticide-treated materials

Insecticide-treated nets may not be appropriate in complex emergency situations where people have no tradition of net use, shelter is very basic, or obtaining sufficient supplies of nets takes a long time or is too costly. In such situations, insecticide treatment of other materials – tents, blankets, sheets, clothing and curtains – may be more acceptable and more feasible. Pyrethroid treatment of these materials has been tried in a range of settings, in particular among Afghan refugees and more recently in Kenya (Macintyre et al., 2003). Some examples are described below. Insecticide-treated blankets and plastic sheeting are the most promising but have not yet passed required WHOPES evaluation. Chapter 8 provides more information about operational research related to insecticide treatment of alternative materials.

Hammock nets

In complex emergency situations where people have to sleep outdoors or in rudimentary shelters, use of hammocks may be an option and mosquito nets that are specially designed for hammocks are available. The feasibility and effectiveness of treating hammock nets with pyrethroid insecticides is currently being evaluated in Cambodia.

Tents

The inner surface of tents can be sprayed using compression sprayers, either in the same way as house spraying or by laying the tent flat before spraying. Tent spraying has been tried with Afghan and Vietnamese refugees, and is carried out each year among nomadic refugees who migrate annually between the Punjab and the mountain areas of Pakistan. In the latter case, tent spraying has been shown to provide 60–80% protection against falciparum malaria (Bouma et al., 1996). The most suitable insecticides for tent spraying are permethrin and deltamethrin, in suspension concentrate (SC) formulation (Hewitt et al., 1995). Wettable powder (WP) formulation, which is used for house spraying, is not suitable for tent spraying. Pyrethroid insecticide persists for more than 12 months on double-sheeted tents and for up to 6 months on single-sheeted tents. A tent made of canvas inter-woven with insecticide-impregnated polyethylene threads has recently been shown to be highly effective against mosquitoes (Graham et al., 2004).

Insecticide-treated plastic sheeting (ITPS)

Research is under way to determine the effectiveness of insecticide treat-ment of the plastic sheeting that is increasingly being provided as shelter in emergencies in Africa (Allan, 2001). The laminated polyethylene tarpaulin is impregnated with deltamethrin during manufacture and the insecticide migrates slowly to the surface to replace that which is lost. Entomological trials in refugee camps in Pakistan showed that the insecticide is present for at least a year and kills mosquitoes that come into contact with it (Graham et al., 2002a). The mode of action of ITPS (approx. size: 4 m x 5 m) would be comparable to indoor residual spraying, with a potential community protective effect at high coverage but no personal protection effect.

Results from an initial field trial in Sierra Leone into the effectiveness of ITPS against malaria are currently being analysed by the Centre for In-ternational Emergency, Disaster and Refugee Studies/Johns Hopkins Uni-versity. The potential of ITPS is likely to depend on local vector resistance patterns and the ratio of ITPS to other mosquito resting sites in a given situ-ation. Evidence from other countries and modes of use (e.g. as roofing, wall, and tent) is still needed. In situations where commercially available ITPS is be-ing used, the duration of effectiveness against malaria, and safety under field conditions should be monitored and reported to build up the evidence base.

Blankets, top sheets and clothing

Permethrin treatment of top sheets, blankets and chaddars (the veil or wrap worn by many Muslim women) has been tried among Afghan refugees. Compared with a placebo, insecticide treatment was shown to provide 62% protection against falciparum malaria and 46% protection against vivax malaria (Rowland et al., 1999). A trial in Kabul, Afghanistan, showed that treated bedding provided a level of protection against cutaneous leishma-niasis (a disease that is transmitted by sandflies) equivalent to that provided by treated nets (Reyburn et al., 2000). Permethrin is the preferred insecti-cide because of its low toxicity, at a target dose of $0.5–1$ g/m^2 (Graham et al., 2002b). The good personal protection afforded by insecticide-treated blankets is due mostly to the repellent effect of the permethrin. Effective-ness is comparable to, but shorter-lived than, that of ITNs.

Treated blankets, top sheets and chaddars could play an important role in malaria prevention in emergencies because they are easily available

– blankets are often included as a standard item in emergency relief kits, and top sheets and chaddars are widely used in some cultures – and because they can be used regardless of whether people sleep indoors or outdoors and of the type of shelter. In addition, providing protection by treating these materials is cheaper than providing protection with treated nets, since the only cost involved is that of the insecticide. The duration of effectiveness of pretreated blankets (either stockpiled or in field use) still needs to be evaluated. Further research is also required to find out whether treated blankets can provide protection against malaria in endemic conditions in Africa: a recent study of permethrin-treated sheets among Kenyan nomads indicates a protective effect (Macintyre et al., 2003) (see also Chapter 8).

Curtains

In areas where mosquitoes bite early in the evening, before people go to sleep under nets, use of insecticide-treated curtains over openings such as windows, doors and eave gaps may provide some protection. Treated curtains can be very cheap if shelters or houses have a limited number of openings. They have been shown to have an impact in some settings, for example in west Africa (Habluetzel et al., 1999) and in Afghanistan, where people have been encouraged to use treated nets as curtains when they move indoors after the summer.

Long-lasting treatment

A number of new long-lasting insecticidal products are expected to reach the market in the near future. Long-lasting formulations that could be used to treat conventional nets in the field may be particularly useful in emergencies, helping to overcome the current delays in supply of long-lasting insecticidal nets, or may be used to improve conventional nets that have already been distributed. It will be important to use products that conform to WHOPES specifications for safety, efficacy and operational acceptability.

Insecticide zooprophylaxis

Insecticide zooprophylaxis could be used in settings where vectors bite domestic animals as well as humans, for example in south and south-west Asia where *A. culicifacies* and *A. stephensi* feed on cattle 90% of the time and humans 10% of the time. Rather than being applied to houses, the insecticide – usually deltamethrin – is applied to the hair and skin of domestic livestock, such as cattle, goats and sheep, using a sponge or animal dip. Mosquitoes pick up a lethal dose of insecticide when they attempt to feed on a "treated" animal.

Trials of this method in Afghan refugee camps have shown its effect on malaria to be comparable to that of IRS but at 20% of the cost, since less insecticide is required (Rowland et al., 2001). Although still at the development stage, insecticide zooprophylaxis has been widely used in Afghan refugee settlements in Pakistan. However, it will not work against anthropophilic vectors such as *A. gambiae* in Africa.

Home-use products

Home-use products include coils, insecticide aerosols, mosquito repellents and vaporizing mats. Like treated curtains, these products may be of some use in areas where mosquitoes bite early in the evening. However, vaporizing mats require electricity, which is unlikely to be available in most resettlement sites or camps.

These methods are needed every evening and may therefore be too costly, although social marketing of mosquito repellents in Afghanistan did have reasonable success and indicated protection against malaria (Rowland et al., 2004a). In acute emergencies repellents may have logistic advantages (e.g. less bulk) over other methods, and a recent trial in an Afghan refugee camp demonstrated up to 50% protective efficacy against falciparum malaria (Rowland et al., 2004b). Repellents may provide a good temporary solution provided that recipients are disciplined about applying them.

Methods that are usually not appropriate in complex emergencies

Larval control

Larval control is most practicable where vector breeding sites are limited in number and relatively permanent. It is thus not feasible in much of rural Africa, where the breeding sites of the major vectors are numerous and temporary, or in south-east Asia, where breeding sites are in inaccessible forest areas. It has not been widely used in complex emergencies and is not advised unless there is professional entomological expertise available to provide support.

In areas where it is a viable option, larval control must be carried out thoroughly if it is to have an impact. The target area must be large enough to include all breeding sites contributing to the local adult mosquito population. Not all water bodies are breeding sites, and many others produce few mosquitoes, so good local knowledge and entomological expertise are required to target the most productive breeding sites. There are three methods of larva control – chemical, biological and environmental.

Chemical methods

Chemical methods of larviciding include the use of oils and chemical and bacterial insecticides.

Few chemical insecticides are safe enough for use in water that is used for drinking and bathing. The most commonly used is the organophosphate temephos, which is effective and safe in drinking-water at a concentration of 1 part per million. In most parts of the world, *Anopheles* species remain fully susceptible to temephos, although resistance is common in nuisance-biting *Culex quinquefasciatus*. Pyrethroid insecticides are highly toxic to fish and are therefore unsuitable in many places.

Bacillus thuringiensis H-14 (BTI), a bacterial insecticide, is specifically toxic to mosquitoes and blackflies. BTI can be very effective but it is costly; moreover, most formulations have a short residual action against surface-feeding *Anopheles*, necessitating weekly re-treatment.

Insecticide can be delivered in dilute liquid form using spray pumps or in granular form. Granular formulations are easier to handle and penetrate better into water that is covered with vegetation.

Biological methods

Biological control is safe but can be difficult to apply, and there are few examples of effective malaria control using biological methods. Fish are the most widely used method, specifically the minnow *Gambusia affinis* and the guppy *Poecilia reticulata*. In an area of Somalia, for example, malaria was controlled successfully by stocking concrete tanks (the only local source of surface water) with larva-eating fish.

Environmental methods

Environmental control methods include removing breeding sites (by filling or draining them) and avoiding the creation of breeding sites. However, good local knowledge and entomological expertise are required to target the most productive breeding sites and to avoid wasting time and resources on unimportant sites.

Scrub removal

There is no evidence that the widely advocated practice of cutting down grass and scrub around houses, to reduce the number of mosquito resting sites, has any impact on malaria transmission.

Aerosol spraying

Outdoor aerosol spraying from a vehicle or using a motorized sprayer looks impressive but there is little evidence that it has any impact on malaria and it is not recommended.

Selecting and implementing prevention methods

Once it is decided that malaria prevention is likely to be useful and feasible, the next consideration is the methods of prevention that are appropriate and how malaria prevention activities can be organized.

Selecting prevention methods

The main criteria for selection of methods of prevention, and the information required for decision-making are:

- *Need* – the burden of malaria; geographical distribution; seasonality; risk of an outbreak.
- *Efficacy* – trials measuring impact; vector prevalence, distribution and behaviour; experience with existing/previous use of ITNs, IRS or other vector control in the area.
- *Effectiveness relative to other malaria control methods* – impact in operational conditions.
- *Costs* – cost-effectiveness; resources; affordability.
- *Feasibility of implementation* – health system logistics and information systems; access to high-risk groups; population movement, behaviour and housing; budget available; availability of human (trained workforce) and material resources; possibilities for supervision and monitoring of activities.

Two of the most difficult decisions to be made are *whether to start* and *when to stop* applying preventive interventions; gathering the information above can guide such decisions. When selecting malaria prevention methods for complex emergencies, it is also important to be aware that emergency situations change. The situation needs to be reviewed on a regular basis, using relevant data, to ensure that prevention methods are still appropriate.

Table 6.3 summarizes the characteristics of malaria in different parts of the world, to help guide selection of appropriate prevention measures.

Organizing malaria prevention activities

Information collected during the initial assessment (see Chapter 2) should be used to plan and organize malaria prevention activities. Additional,

Table 6.3 **Characteristics of different malaria situations and possible actions required**

Epidemiological type	Characteristics of malaria	Possible prevention activities
Savannah or grassland (sub-Saharan Africa, Papua New Guinea)	• Generally present throughout the year • Seasonal increase • Drug resistance, mainly *P. falciparum* • Affects mainly children and pregnant women	• Insecticide-treated mosquito nets • Other types of personal protection • Health promotion
Plains and valleys outside Africa (Central America, China, Indian subcontinent)	• Moderate transmission • Often mainly *P. vivax* • Major seasonal variation • Risk of outbreaks	• Spraying of houses • Insecticide-treated mosquito nets • Other types of personal protection • Livestock treatment • Health promotion
Highland and desert fringe (African and south-east Asian highlands, Sahel, southern Africa, south-west Pacific)	• High risk of outbreaks • Major seasonal variation • Influenced by agricultural practices • Migration may lead to outbreaks	• Spraying of houses may be considered • Localized house spraying for prevention of outbreaks • Insecticide-treated mosquito nets • Health promotion
Urban and peri-urban (Africa, South America, south Asia)	• Highly variable transmission • Immunity of the population variable • Specially adapted urban vectors responsible for outbreaks in south Asia	• Insecticide-treated mosquito nets • Other personal protection • Control of breeding sites by larviciding or environmental planning and management • Spraying of houses in selected areas • Health promotion
Forest and forest fringe (south-east Asia, South America)	• Focal intense transmission • Many risk groups, often occupational	• Insecticide-treated mosquito nets • Other personal protection • Consider siting of dwellings • Health promotion

more specific, information, for example about each particular site, may be needed to guide the organization and monitoring of activities. Table 6.4 shows how information about the population, vectors and environment can be used in the organization of malaria prevention activities.

Important steps in setting up prevention activities are:

1. Collect information (epidemiological, demographic, logistic, etc.) from local experts.
2. Choose sites for camps and rehousing of people away from vector breeding sites.
3. Define control objectives based on the severity of the problem, available resources and the level of health care in the area or host country.
4. Choose control measures.
5. Identify possible local suppliers. In selecting suppliers, keep cost and quality in mind – sometimes an international supplier may be preferable.
6. Identify appropriate agencies to implement programmes.
7. Plan a training programme for local staff.
8. Implement the chosen control measures.
9. Monitor and evaluate control measures in terms of cost-effectiveness and quality.

Mosquito life-cycle, behaviour and biological features

For the purposes of vector control, it is important to:

— understand the life-cycle and natural history of mosquitoes;
— be able to recognize different types of mosquito;
— understand mosquito behaviour; and
— know the susceptibility of mosquitoes to insecticides.

The mosquito life-cycle

There are four main stages in the life-cycle of the mosquito – egg, larva, pupa and adult.

- *Egg.* Mosquitoes lay eggs on water in batches of 70–200 every few days. *Anopheles* eggs are about 0.5 mm long and float on the surface of water for 2–3 days until they hatch; unlike *Aedes* eggs, they cannot survive if they dry out.

- *Larva.* Each egg hatches into a larva, which swims and feeds. *Anopheles* larvae float horizontally on the surface of the water, whereas *Aedes* and *Culex* larvae hang down into the water with just their breathing tubes at

Table 6.4 **Using information to plan and organize malaria prevention activities**

Type of information	Why is this information important?	How can this information be used?
Environment		
• Climate, rainfall, surface water, temperature, vegetation, topography	Affects potential for transmission	To determine mosquito control strategies and predict outbreaks.
Host		
• Population size	Indicates the total number of people at risk.	To plan amount of supplies needed.
• Distribution	Indicates accessibility of people, urban and rural environment.	To determine the type of malaria control activities required.
• Mobility	Increases possibility of outbreaks.	
• Types of dwellings and location in relation to breeding sites	Open dwellings are difficult to spray. Different types of dwellings need different net designs. Proximity of breeding sites increases risk.	
• Night-time behaviour	If people are outside during the mosquito biting time, their risk of infection is higher.	To protect children by suggesting when they should be protected by a net.
Vector		
• Species	Different species have different behaviours.	To influence mosquito control strategy.
• Preferred breeding sites	Indicates which water bodies are important and whether larval control is feasible.	To help determine control methods and communication messages.
• Resting habits (inside, outside)	House spraying and insecticide-treated nets may be more effective against indoor-resting vectors.	
• Feeding habits (time, host preference, location)	House spraying and insecticide-treated nets may be more effective against indoor biters and if people are inside at peak biting time.	To help determine control methods and communication messages.
• Seasonal density changes	Affects seasonal pattern of disease.	To help determine content of communication messages and timing of control activities.

the surface. As the larvae grow to full size (about 1 cm long) they shed their skin four times. In the tropics, mosquitoes can complete the larval stage in only 7 days.

- *Pupa*. The larva develops into a pupa, which is shaped like a comma. The pupa does not feed but comes to the surface of the water to breathe. The pupa stage lasts 2–3 days.

- *Adult*. The adult mosquito that emerges from the pupa has three main parts – head, thorax and abdomen. The head has eyes, antennae, palps and mouth parts or proboscis. Only the female mosquito feeds on blood. The easiest way to distinguish male from female mosquitoes is by looking at the antennae, which are feathery in males.

Adult mosquitoes mate soon after emerging from the pupae. In most species, the female can produce eggs only after feeding on blood from a human or animal. Once the blood-meal is digested and the eggs have developed, the female mosquito finds a suitable place to lay the eggs. This 2–3-day cycle of feeding, developing and laying eggs is called the gonotrophic cycle and it is repeated throughout the remaining life of the adult female mosquito.

In favourable conditions, female adult mosquitoes live an average of 10–14 days, although some live much longer. The lifespan of the male adult mosquito is shorter. The lifespan of the female is most important in malaria transmission, since it takes at least 10 days for the malaria parasites in the mosquito to become infective to humans; thus, only mosquitoes that live longer than this will be able to transmit malaria. Factors that affect the lifespan of the adult mosquito include temperature, humidity, natural enemies, and vector control measures. Where temperatures exceed 35 °C and the humidity is less than 50%, mosquitoes die much sooner.

Different types of mosquito

Malaria is transmitted by *Anopheles* mosquitoes. Some *Anopheles* mosquitoes can also carry other human diseases, such as filariasis (elephantiasis). *Aedes* mosquitoes are important vectors of yellow fever and dengue and *Culex* mosquitoes of filariasis and Japanese encephalitis. There are three main ways to distinguish *Anopheles* mosquitoes from culicine mosquitoes such as *Aedes*, *Culex* and *Mansonia* (see Table 6.5). The differences in each stage of the life cycle of *Anopheles*, *Aedes* and *Culex* mosquitoes are shown in Figure 6.1.

Table 6.5 **Three ways to distinguish anopheline from culicine mosquitoes**
(see also Figure 6.1)

Characteristic	Anophelines	Culicines
Resting position	Normally rest at an angle to the surface.	Normally rest with the body parallel to the surface.
Wings	Appear to have black and white spots, because the dark and pale scales on the wings are arranged in blocks.	Do not appear to have black and white spots.
Palps (in female mosquitoes)	Are the same length as the proboscis.	Are only a third of the length of the proboscis.

Mosquito behaviour

Several aspects of mosquito behaviour are relevant for vector control – resting location, feeding time and location, host preference, flight range and choice of egg laying site.

Resting location

After feeding, a female adult mosquito needs somewhere to rest while she digests the blood and develops the eggs. Some species remain inside, while others go and find resting places outdoors. It is easier to control vectors that rest indoors with residual spraying in houses; for example, this method is used to control the indoor-resting vectors A. *culicifacies* and A. *stephensi* in the Indian subcontinent.

Feeding time and location

Most *Anopheles* feed at night – each species feeds at a particular time of night. For example, A. *farauti* in the Solomon Islands and A. *maculatus* near the Thai–Myanmar border bite as soon as it is dark and feed mostly in the early evening; by contrast, A. *gambiae* in Africa and A. *dirus* in southeast Asia feed late at night.

Some mosquitoes prefer to feed inside houses and others outside. It is easier to use residual spraying of houses to control vectors that feed indoors and ITNs for vectors that feed outside. However, residual spraying is useful for species that feed outside and then enter houses to rest, such as A. *culicifacies* in Pakistan.

Host preference

Some mosquito species prefer to feed on humans and others on animals; several species feed partly on humans and partly on animals. Species that

Figure 6.1 **The life-cycles of *Anopheles*, *Aedes* and *Culex* mosquitoes**[a]

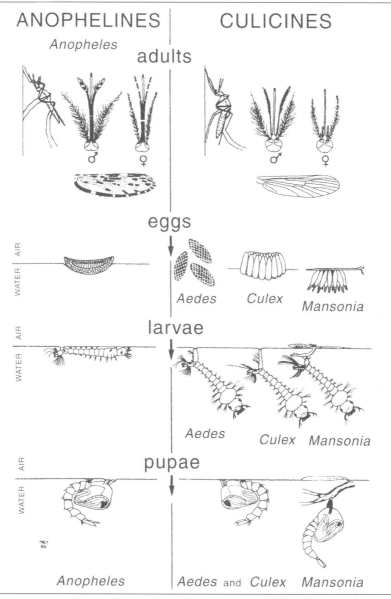

[a] Source: Warrell DA, Gilles HM, eds. *Essential malariology*, 4th ed. London, Hodder Arnold, 2002. Reproduced by kind permission of the publisher.

have a strong preference for feeding on humans, for example *A. gambiae* in Africa, tend to be the most dangerous vectors because they are the most likely to pick up and pass on malaria parasites.

Flight range

Most *Anopheles* mosquitoes do not fly more than 3 km from where they begin their lives. Malaria risk can be reduced by siting refugee camps further than 3 km from breeding sites.

Choice of egg laying site

Anopheles mosquitoes have different preferences for breeding sites or larval habitats, and lay their eggs in a wide variety of water bodies. However, individual species tend to choose a narrow range of egg laying sites.

Insecticide susceptibility

Mosquitoes that become resistant to a particular insecticide (see Box 6.5) are less likely to be controlled by that insecticide. However, even when resistance is detected in a species, it may be unnecessary to change the insecticide or the vector control method: if the resistance frequency is low (only a minority of mosquitoes carry resistance) or the resistance is weak, the insecticide might still be used to good effect. Resistant mosquitoes that have lived long enough to incubate malaria parasites to maturity sometimes become less resistant as they grow older and hence more vulnerable to insecticide residues. There is evidence from west Africa that insecticide-treated nets continue to be protective against pyrethroid-resistant *A. gambiae* (Corbel, 2004), whereas IRS with pyrethroids has lost effectiveness against resistant *A. funestus* in South Africa, necessitating a return to DDT spraying (Hargreaves et al., 2000). If the insecticide or vector control method is

Box 6.5 **Development of insecticide resistance**

A species of mosquito that is exposed to an insecticide for many generations may develop physiological resistance to that type of insecticide. This is an evolutionary (Darwinian) process in which mosquitoes that carry genes for resistance survive exposure to insecticide and pass on these genes to the next generation of mosquitoes. The gene for resistance arises initially by mutation. Selection of mosquitoes resistant to DDT was one of the reasons for the failure of malaria eradication efforts in the 1950s and 1960s. In some regions, resistance has since developed to other types of insecticide, including malathion and other organophosphates, and pyrethroids.

no longer achieving the same level of malaria control it should be changed. (Chapter 8 gives more information about detecting resistance.) Tables 6.6–6.9 summarize the relevant biological features of some of the most important vectors in south-east Asia, Africa, south Asia and South America.

Table 6.6 **Significant biological features of major and some minor malaria vectors in Cambodia, Lao People's Democratic Republic, Myanmar, Thailand and Viet Nam**[a]

Anopheles species	Resting location	Feeding time and location	Host preferences	Breeding sites	Insecticide susceptibility
A. dirus complex (7 sibling species; described as A. balabacensis in earlier literature)	Mainly outside	Mainly late (or 20:00– 02:00 hrs) Outside and inside	Mainly human	Small shady pools mainly in forests and plantations, footprints, stream seepages, wheel ruts, gem pits, hollow logs, sometimes wells	Susceptible to DDT and others
A. minimus (at least 2 sibling species)	Mainly outside (previously inside)	All night Mainly outside (previously inside)	Human and cows	Streams in forested foothills	Susceptible to DDT
A. maculatus complex (8 sibling species)	Mainly outside	Peak 19:00– 20:00 or 21:00– 24.00 hrs Mainly outside	Mainly non-human	Sunlit streams, sometimes ponds, tanks, riverbed pools	Susceptible to DDT and others
A. sundaicus (2 sibling species suspected)	Outside and inside	All night, peak 20:00– 24:00 hrs Outside and inside	Human and domestic animals	Brackish or salt water near coast, rock pools, river mouths	DDT resistance in Indonesia and Viet Nam

[a] Source: Meek (1995). Reproduced by kind permission of the publisher.

Table 6.7 **Significant biological features of major malaria vectors in Africa**[a]

Anopheles species	Resting location	Feeding time and location	Host preferences	Breeding sites	Insecticide susceptibility
A. gambiae	Mainly inside	Mainly late Inside	Mainly humans	Sunlit temporary pools, rice fields	Resistance to DDT, HCH,[b] recently to pyrethroids in west Africa
A. arabiensis	Inside and outside	Mainly late Inside and outside	Humans and animals	Temporary pools, rice fields	Resistance to DDT, and to malathion in Sudan
A. melas	Outside and inside	Mainly late Inside and outside	Animals and humans	Saltwater lagoons, mangrove swamps	
A. merus	Outside and inside	Mainly late Inside and outside	Mainly animals	Saltwater lagoons, mangrove swamps	
A. funestus	Inside	Mainly late Inside	Mainly humans	Semipermanent and permanent water, especially with vegetation, swamps, slow streams, ditch edges	Resistance to DDT, recently to pyrethroids in southern Africa

[a] Source: Mehra (1995).
[b] Hexachlorocyclohexane.

Table 6.8 **Significant biological features of major malaria vectors in south Asia**

Anopheles species	Resting location	Feeding time and location	Host preferences	Breeding sites	Insecticide susceptibility
A. stephensi (urban "type" and rural "mysorensis" forms)	Mainly inside	Late evening and night Inside and outside	Mainly cattle and domestic animals	Urban vector: domestic water tanks and containers, construction sites Rural vector: borrow pits, river margins, rice fields	Resistant to DDT, HCH,[a] malathion
A. culicifacies (5 sibling species of differing vectoral capacity)	Mainly inside	Late evening and night Inside and outside	Mainly cattle and domestic animals	Rural vector: clean water, river margins, rice fields, manmade pits and pools	Resistant to DDT, HCH,[a] malathion

[a] Hexachlorocyclohexane.

Table 6.9 **Significant biological features of major malaria vectors in South America**

Anopheles species	Resting location	Feeding time and location	Host preferences	Breeding sites	Insecticide susceptibility
A. albimanus (Central America to northern South America)	Mostly outside, some inside – for control IRS is standard but ITNs shown to be effective in Nicaragua	Late evening Inside	Domestic animals (cattle, horses), 80% humans 20%	Stagnant water, flooded pasture, or water with 25% emergent vegetation coverage	Broad-spectrum resistance to organophosphates and carbamates (low level), pyrethroids and DDT
A. darlingi (Brazil to Mexico)	Inside and outside – for control IRS (DDT and lambdacy-halothrin) and ITNs	Throughout the night, but with biting peaks at dusk and dawn. Mainly inside	Humans	Breeding sites and epidemics associated with deforestation and mining	Some DDT resistance
A. aquasalis (coastal areas from east Venezuela to south Brazil)	Outside – not controlled by IRS	Late at night Outside	Mainly domestic animals (cattle, horses, pigs)	Brackish water, mangrove, temporary freshwater	

References

Allan R (2001). Roll Back Malaria – facing the challenges in complex emergencies. *The Health Exchange*, 5 December, 4–8.

Bouma M et al. (1996). Malaria control using permethrin applied to tents of nomadic Afghan refugees in northern Pakistan. *Bulletin of the World Health Organization*, 74:413–421.

Cong LD, Schapira A (1998). The will to win in Viet Nam. *World Health*, 51(3):27.

Corbel V et al. (2004). Dosage-dependent effects of permethrin-treated nets on the behaviour of *Anopheles gambiae* and the selection of pyrethroid resistance. *Malaria Journal*, 3:22.

Graham K et al. (2002a). Insecticide treated plastic tarpaulins for control of malaria vectors in refugee camps. *Medical and Veterinary Entomology*, 16:404–408.

Graham K et al. (2002b). Comparison of three pyrethroid treatments of top-sheets for malaria control in emergencies: entomological and user acceptance studies in an Afghan refugee camp in Pakistan. *Medical and Veterinary Entomology*, 16:199–207.

Graham K et al. (2004). Tents pre-treated with insecticide for malaria control in refugee camps: an entomological evaluation. *Malaria Journal*, 3: 25.

Graham K et al. (2005). Multi-country trials comparing wash resistance of PermaNet and conventional insecticide treated nets against anopheline and culicine mosquitoes. *Medical and Veterinary Entomology*, 19: 72–83.

Habluetzel A et al. (1999). Insecticide-treated curtains reduce the prevalence and intensity of malaria infection in Burkina Faso. *Tropical Medicine and International Health*, 4:557–564.

Hargreaves K et al. (2000). *Anopheles funestus* resistant to pyrethroid insecticides in South Africa. *Medical and Veterinary Entomology*, 14: 181–189.

Hewitt S et al. (1995). Pyrethroid sprayed tents for malaria control: an entomological evaluation in Pakistan. *Medical and Veterinary Entomology*, 9:344–352.

Luxemburger C et al. (1996). The epidemiology of malaria in a Karen population on the western border of Thailand. *Transactions of the Royal Society of Tropical Medicine and Hygiene*, 90:105–111.

Macintyre K et al. (2003). A new tool for malaria prevention? Results of a trial of permethrin-impregnated bedsheets (shukas) in an area of unstable transmission. *International Journal of Epidemiology*, 32:157–160.

Meek SR (1995). Vector control in some countries of South-east Asia: comparing the vectors and the strategies. *Annals of Tropical Medicine and Parasitology*, 89:135–147.

Mehra S et al. (1995). *Partnerships for change and communication: guidelines for malaria control*. Geneva, World Health Organization.

Reyburn H et al. (2000). A randomised controlled trial of insecticide-treated bednets and chaddars or top sheets, and residual spraying or interior rooms for the prevention of cutaneous leishmaniasis in Kabul, Afghanistan. *Transactions of the Royal Society of Tropical Medicine and Hygiene*, 94:361–366.

Rowland M et al. (1997). Sustainability of pyrethroid-impregnated bed nets for malaria control in Afghan communities. *Bulletin of the World Health Organization*, 75:23–29.

Rowland M et al. (1999). Permethrin-treated chaddars and top-sheets: appropriate technology for protection against malaria in Afghanistan and other complex emergencies. *Transactions of the Royal Society of Tropical Medicine and Hygiene*, 93:465–472.

Rowland M et al. (2001). Control of malaria in Pakistan by applying deltamethrin insecticide to cattle: a community-randomised trial. *Lancet*, 357:1837–1841.

Rowland M et al. (2004a). DEET mosquito repellent sold through social marketing provides protection against malaria in an area of all-night mosquito biting and partial coverage of insecticide-treated nets: a case-control study of effectiveness. *Tropical Medicine and International Health*, 9:343–350.

Rowland M et al. (2004b). DEET mosquito repellent provides personal protection against malaria: a household randomized trial in an Afghan refugee camp in Pakistan. *Tropical Medicine and International Health*, 9:335–342.

Rozendaal JA (1997). *Vector control: methods for use by individuals and communities*. Geneva, World Health Organization.

WHO (2000). *Manual for indoor residual spraying: application of residual sprays for vector control*. Geneva, World Health Organization (WHO/CDS/WHOPES/GCDPP/2000.3 Rev.1).

Further reading

Chavasse D et al. (1999). *Insecticide-treated mosquito nets: a handbook for managers.* London, Malaria Consortium.

Chavasse DC, Yap HH, eds (1997). *Chemical methods for the control of vectors and pests of public health importance.* Geneva, World Health Organization (WHO/CTD/WHOPES/97.2).

Curtis CF, ed. (1991). *Control of disease vectors in the community.* London, Wolfe.

Warrell DA, Gilles HM, eds (2002). *Essential malariology*, 4th ed. London, Arnold.

Matthews GA (2000). *Pesticide application methods*, 3rd ed. Oxford, Blackwell Science.

Nájera JA (1996). *Malaria control among refugees and displaced populations.* Geneva, World Health Organization (CTD/MAL/96.6).

Nájera JA, Zaim M (2002). *Malaria vector control: decision making criteria and procedures for judicious use of insecticides.* Geneva, World Health Organization (WHO/CDS/WHOPES/2002.5 Rev.1).

PAHO (1982). *Emergency vector control after natural disasters.* Washington, DC, Pan American Health Organization.

Sabatinelli G (1997). *Vector and pest control in refugee situations.* Geneva, United Nations High Commissioner for Refugees.

Service MM (1986). *Lecture notes on medical entomology.* Oxford, Blackwell Science.

Thomson MC (1995). *Disease prevention through vector control: guidelines for relief organisations.* Oxford, Oxfam.

WHO (1982). *Manual on environmental management for mosquito control, with special emphasis on malaria vectors.* Geneva, World Health Organization (WHO offset publication no. 66).

WHO (1992a). *Entomological field techniques for malaria control. Part 1. Learner's guide.* Geneva, World Health Organization.

WHO (1992b). *Entomological field techniques for malaria control. Part 2. Tutor's guide.* Geneva, World Health Organization.

WHO (1993). *Equipment for vector control.* Geneva, World Health Organization.

WHO/RBM website: http://www.who.int/malaria.

Finding out more

Malaria in Emergencies Network
World Health Organization
1211 Geneva 27
Switzerland
Fax: +41 22 791 4824
E-mail: rbmemergencies@who.int

Dr Sylvia Meek, Technical Director
Malaria Consortium
Development House
56–64 Leonard Street,
London EC2A 4JX
England
Tel: +44 20 7549 0210 (7549 0214 direct)
Fax: +44 20 7549 0211
E-mail: s.meek@malariaconsortium.org
Web site: www.malariaconsortium.org

Mark Rowland
Department of Infectious Diseases
London School of Hygiene & Tropical Medicine
Keppel Streel
London WC1E 7HT
England
Tel: +44 20 7299 4719
Fax:+44 20 7299 4720
E-mail: mark.rowland@lshtm.ac.uk

CHAPTER 7

Community participation and health education

This chapter:
- outlines guiding principles for community participation and health education related to malaria control in complex emergencies
- describes how to involve communities in malaria control activities, including health education
- identifies specific issues to consider when planning and implementing health education related to malaria control.

Community participation and health education in complex emergencies

Community participation and health education are often seen as being of low priority in complex emergencies, and there is little published information describing practical field experience of these areas of activity. However, there is growing recognition that community participation and health education are essential to the success of malaria control interventions in emergency situations (see Box 7.1), and that more attention should be paid to understanding community perspectives and the sociocultural factors that influence the behaviour of communities and emergency partners (Médecins Sans Frontières, 1997; Williams, 2001; Bloland & Williams, 2003).

The following guiding principles are important both for effective community participation and for health education related to malaria control in complex emergencies:

- Establish mechanisms that promote good communication and enable representatives of the displaced or affected population, the host population, and local and international emergency partners to participate in malaria control.
- Find out about the affected communities.
- Work together with community and organizational representatives to agree on priority needs and to decide what interventions are needed to address these needs.

Box 7.1 **Importance of community participation and health education in malaria control**

Community involvement and effective health education play a critical role in both treatment-seeking and malaria prevention.

Malaria treatment-seeking
The effectiveness of case management depends to some extent on community understanding and action. One of the reasons for high malaria mortality in both emergency and non-emergency situations is late presentation of cases to, or failure to seek treatment from, health facilities. Communities need to be able to recognize the signs of malaria illness and seek effective treatment promptly.

Malaria prevention
The effectiveness of most prevention methods also depends on community understanding and action. Communities need to know why the use of insecticide-treated nets (ITNs) is important and to ensure that young children and pregnant women sleep under treated nets, and community cooperation is essential for indoor residual spraying (IRS) of insecticides.

- Ensure that the community is involved in collecting information and in planning and implementing malaria control activities. Community involvement can also ensure that communication activities and health education methods are socially and culturally appropriate.
- Involve community and organizational representatives in monitoring and evaluating activities.

Before community participation or health education activities are started, it is also important to collect baseline data. This can be done through a rapid ethnographic assessment. Such an assessment can provide information about, for example, the demographics of the population at risk, local terms used to describe malaria, community structures and social norms (see also Chapter 8).

Promoting community participation
Establishing good communication
Good communication is essential if different organizations and community representatives are to work together effectively. Communication between the various emergency partners working in a complex emergency (see Chapter 1) is as important as communication between these organizations and the affected populations.

A working group should be set up at the start of a complex emergency to promote good communication between representatives of emergency partners, local agencies and the affected population, and to ensure effective planning and coordination of malaria control activities. The working group should involve:

— all agencies – including international organizations and NGOs – working in malaria control activities, for example case management, vector control, health education, water and sanitation;
— camp or resettlement officials;
— representatives of UNHCR and other United Nations agencies;
— representatives of the displaced or refugee population, including camp leaders, community elders, block or sector leaders, community committees;
— representatives of the host population and government.

The working group should meet regularly; it is critical that everyone involved agree on malaria control priorities and strategies and the role that the different representatives and organizations will play. The working group should also communicate its activities to other organizations providing health care. This is particularly important where resources are limited because interventions can be planned that address several issues simultaneously – for example, the use of ITNs to prevent both malaria and other mosquito-transmitted diseases.

The active participation of community representatives in the working group is essential for effective communication of information from emergency partners to the community and vice versa (Rifkin, 1996). This helps to ensure that agencies are aware of, and address, community priorities – which will help to give people a sense of being in control of their lives. Without good communication there is a risk that the community will not support malaria control interventions because it has different priorities; there is also a risk that agencies remain unaware of local beliefs and behaviours that may have an impact on malaria control interventions or that the community will fail to appreciate why these interventions are important. Professionals need to listen to the perspectives of those with less formal education and training, and to recognize that communities have their own knowledge and beliefs that can help or hinder malaria control activities.

The first example in Box 7.2 illustrates the importance of giving community leaders an opportunity to express their concerns and of understanding these concerns. Good communication is also important to prevent misunderstanding: in the second example, the desired behaviour change did not

BOX 7.2 **Importance of good communication with the community**

Community concerns about research

In an African refugee camp, drug efficacy studies were planned for children under 5 years old. To ensure that this was acceptable to the community, meetings were held with camp officials, community health workers and refugee leaders. One of the major concerns was why the studies included only children aged less than 5 years when adults were also suffering from malaria. Once it was explained that children are particularly vulnerable and that appropriate treatment for children would also benefit the adult population, community leaders agreed to support the research, and messages were sent out to the residential blocks encouraging people to participate if they were asked to.

Community fears about "breaking the contract"

In another African refugee camp, an agency introduced an ITN programme, attempting to distribute one net to each household. To help with future monitoring and evaluation, the agency stencilled its logo onto each net (so that they could determine whether nets were being traded outside the camp) and asked each household head to sign what appeared to be a formal "contract" stating that the nets had been received. When agency representatives visited the households some weeks later, they were surprised to find that the nets were not being used. The reason was that the monitoring and evaluation measures were perceived by some households to be highly intimidating. Fear of "breaking the contract'" if there were any damage to the nets meant that families were keeping the nets in good condition in their wrappers rather than using them for the intended purpose.

occur because the community did not understand, and was intimidated by, the measures an agency introduced for future monitoring and evaluation.

Understanding the community

Social factors (structures and organization) and cultural factors (language, beliefs and behaviours that are common to a group of people) play an important role in malaria control. To be able to promote effective community participation it is important to find out about the social and cultural context of the displaced or refugee population and of the host community. It is also important to understand the "culture" of the "humanitarian relief community".

- *The displaced or refugee community.* Within the displaced or refugee population there may be numerous subgroups that are socially and culturally diverse and have different priorities. For example, each subgroup may have its own ideas about the causes and treatment of malaria and will interpret health education messages in different ways. The displaced or refugee population may or may not share the same culture as the host community. This can influence the attitudes and perceptions of the host community towards the displaced or refugee population.

- *The host community.* It is important to understand the social and cultural context of the host community in order to address its needs; this is especially true of a host community living close to camps or resettlement areas. Providing services for the displaced or refugee population that are not available to the host community can cause hostility and conflict (see Chapter 1).

- *The "humanitarian relief community".* The different organizations working in an emergency situation – local and government agencies, international organizations, and NGOs – may share many values and beliefs but may also have different perspectives and priorities. Successful coordination depends on understanding and recognizing these differences (Watson, 1999).

For both the displaced or refugee population and the host population, it is essential to understand how social organization has been changed by the emergency situation (see Table 7.1), and to be aware that structures similar to those that existed before the emergency will rapidly begin to develop. It is particularly important to:

- Find out about social organization, the roles that are played by different groups and individuals, and who influences attitudes and behaviours. Learning how residential units are organized will provide information about the social structure, for example, block leaders, and about any political divisions that might affect implementation of control activities.

- Be sensitive to people's need to regain control, self-determination, and a sense of meaning to their lives.

- Identify all vulnerable groups – not only those that are physiologically vulnerable to malaria, such as pregnant women and young children, but also those that may be vulnerable for political, ethnic, social or cultural reasons. Minority groups, for example, may be politically vulnerable and so unable to access health facilities or to participate fully in community education or prevention activities.

Table 7.1 **Comparing community organization before and after displacement**[a]

	Before	After
Formal organizations	• Government and social service agencies	• May be absent or centred around political, ethnic or religious groups
Semi-formal organizations	• Schools	• Schools (in later phases)
	• Religious organizations	• Religious organizations (in later phases); religious leaders may be a significant presence in all phases of an emergency
	• Neighbourhoods	• Residential units not organized; in later phases residential blocks develop and block leaders emerge
	• Social organizations	• Social organizations; in later phases may develop as grassroots approach to meeting community needs
Opinion leaders	• May be formal or informal	• May be formal or informal; community health workers may play this role initially
Family, kin and social networks	• Family, kin and social networks	• May be widely dispersed, normal channels of advice and support may be lacking; ad hoc networks may be formed by individuals who fled together

[a] Person & Cotton, 1996.

Working with the community to identify priority needs and activities

Priorities should be based on community needs and perspectives, but will also depend on the resources that are available to agencies and on what can be achieved in the local context. In the acute phase of an emergency, however, there may be immediate needs, such as dealing with a malaria outbreak, which are often determined by health professionals. Once the situation stabilizes, community priorities and other activities, such as prevention, can be given more attention.

Involving the community in defining priority needs and activities (see Box 7.3) can improve the effectiveness of malaria control activities. To do this, it may be helpful to adapt existing guidelines for community participation in malaria control (Meek, 1995) for use in emergency situations (see also "Further reading" at the end of this chapter).

Collecting information

Individuals recruited from the displaced or refugee population can be used to help collect information about the community and priority needs. They

Box 7.3 **Involving the community**

- Find out how to show respect to community leaders.
- Listen to the concerns of the displaced or refugee and host populations.
- Allow community representatives to define their own concerns and priorities first. This is important because people in some cultures will agree with those they perceive to be more powerful, even if they do not support the idea or what is being said – and community agreement to proposals from international agencies may therefore not be what it seems.
- Define together the problems, their causes and the possible solutions.
- Involve community representatives in planning and implementing qualitative research to gather information, and in analysing the data collected (see "Collecting information" below).
- Relate malaria control activities to local ideas about cause, symptoms and cure. If feasible, involve traditional healers in case management and referral.
- Provide clear information about how and where malaria control activities will take place; for example, specify the location of clinics and outreach centres, the timing and location of spraying, net distribution and treatment. If possible, involve community representatives in carrying out prevention measures such as spraying, net distribution and re-treatment.
- Be sensitive to gender and ethnicity. Be aware that community leaders may not represent the views of women, the most vulnerable, or minority groups in the affected population. Try to include representatives from these groups. For example, link malaria control to the activities of women's groups or programmes that target women: in several refugee camps in the United Republic of Tanzania, the Tanzanian Red Cross used women's groups to sew mosquito nets, and this contributed both to controlling malaria and to generating income for women.

share a common language and culture with the population, which can greatly facilitate communication. They can also provide useful and specific information, for example about community leadership, structure and politics. It is important to be aware that initial contact will often be with the most educated and influential people and that efforts will therefore be needed to collect information from other subgroups who may not be represented by community leaders. Box 7.4 provides general guidelines for use when gathering community-level information during a research study or evaluation exercise.

One way to learn about the community and to identify vulnerable subgroups is to walk through the residential units of a camp or resettlement area with community members.

- Do not walk with the most visible or important leaders, as community members may be reluctant to voice concerns in front of these leaders or

Box 7.4 **Collecting information from the community**

■ Gather information about specific topics from key informants or focus groups.

■ Choose key informants carefully. They should be individuals who are well known to the community, understand the information needed, and can communicate freely with you and interpret the information in a culturally meaningful way. Be aware that key informants may not be representative of the majority of the community.

■ Include community members in research or evaluation teams when possible. This makes it easier to work with the community and also provides additional insights during information gathering and analysis.

■ Give feedback on your findings to the community during the information-gathering process, so that you can adjust questions and methods if necessary.

■ Involve the community in developing recommendations.

■ Continue community participatory research during the implementation of malaria control activities to improve their effectiveness.

to reveal what is happening in their residential units. Community health workers or trusted volunteers are more appropriate for community walks.

- Walk through the community at randomly chosen times of the day, on several different days and in different areas.

- Do not tell the community of your visit in advance. In this way, people will be engaged in typical daily activities rather than preparing for a "guest". However, if an unannounced visit violates cultural ideas of politeness or poses a security risk, community leaders should be alerted about the timing and purpose of the visit.

- During the walk, stop and hold informal conversations with community members. Ask them about the community – who is in need of what services, who has been sick recently or who is frequently sick. This approach will help to provide information about less obvious community dynamics, which some leaders may be reluctant to discuss.

- Try to take notes as you walk, recording the actual behaviours and situations that you see, as well as what people tell you.

To identify priorities, it is also essential to collect answers from the community to the following questions:

- What is their previous experience with malaria control activities?
- What malaria control activities are in place?

- What do they think and do about febrile illnesses, including malaria?
- What local words and terms are used to describe malaria?
- What does the community believe about the causes, symptoms and treatment of malaria?
- What sources of information are used and trusted by the community?
- When and where do people seek treatment for malaria?
- What does the community do to prevent malaria?
- What are the community's priorities for malaria control?
- What factors would encourage the community to take prevention measures and to seek treatment?
- What factors might stop the community from taking prevention measures or seeking treatment?

This information can be collected using qualitative methods, which focus on learning about what is important to the community. Box 7.5 summarizes different qualitative methods. If possible, a social scientist should be employed to help design qualitative research tools and collect information; alternatively, local experts can be consulted. However, if time and resources are limited, rapid assessment techniques may have to be used to collect this information (see references and "Further reading" at the end of this chapter). Chapter 8 and Annex VII include examples of questions that can be asked to guide the development of malaria control activities.

Involving the community in implementation

The affected community is a partner in, not the target of, control activities, and individuals who are well known and trusted by the community must be involved in implementation. It is important to consider how a cadre of community "activists" can be developed and how community organizations – women's groups, centres of worship, etc. – can be used to mobilize others to participate in malaria control activities.

Community members and community health workers can play an important role in a range of malaria control activities, including the following.

- *Case management* – for example, involving traditional healers in the work of the clinic (see Box 7.6), or training community health workers to carry out surveillance for suspected malaria cases and to supervise treatment with antimalarials. In the United Republic of Tanzania, community health workers were assigned the task of visiting all the homes in their residential blocks to ensure that malaria patients had taken chloroquine correctly during the 3-day treatment period. Community

Box 7.5 **Qualitative methods**

■ *Individual interviews* – are guided by a mixture of structured and open-ended questions to explore topics related to malaria control. People to be interviewed can either be selected purposively (that is, with a specific reason or topic in mind), e.g. as key informants, community leaders or health workers, or be selected randomly. An advantage of individual interviews is that questions can be flexibly structured and related topics raised by the person being interviewed can be pursued.

■ *Focus group discussions* – involve discussions with groups of 8–15 people with similar backgrounds. A facilitator guides the discussion using a checklist of questions or topics; a second person records what participants say and notes how they interact. Focus group discussions are a useful initial method for finding out what topics are important to people. They can also be used to clarify or check information collected during individual interviews.

■ *Free listing* – a method that involves people being asked to list as many different aspects as possible of the topic of interest. For example, the question "What methods are used in this community to prevent malaria?" can generate a wealth of information that can be used to develop questions for interviews or topics for focus group discussions, as well as to guide the design of malaria control interventions. An advantage of free listing is that it provides a large amount of information in a short period of time – and can be carried out, for example, in the form of a game.

■ *Pile sorting* – uses information identified through free listing to find out how people perceive and make sense of various issues. Individuals or groups are asked to sort the issues they have listed into categories. For Example, asking them to sort a list of malaria treatments into categories that make sense to them may provide information about the remedies people use for different types of malaria. This information can help with the design of interventions.

■ *Mapping* – uses maps drawn by community members to show different community features, such as where clinics are located or where malaria is a particular problem. Mapping provides useful information about community perspectives on their situation.

■ *Venn diagram* – a participatory method that provides information about the social structure of a population, for example identifying community leaders and people with influence, and about the relationships between the community and outside agencies. This information can help to identify who might support or oppose malaria control activities.

members were also used as peer role models to improve case management (see Box 7.7).

- *Prevention measures* – for example, training community members as community health educators (see Box 7.8) or in the manufacture and repair of mosquito nets, or involving them in insecticide spraying or in setting up net distribution or re-treatment systems (see Box 7.9).

- *Epidemiology* – for example, training local health workers to interpret the routine information they collect to help in designing malaria control interventions (see Box 7.8).

- *Environmental control* – for example, participation of community members in sanitation improvements, design of irrigation schemes, establishing biological control methods.

Box 7.6 **Involving traditional healers in case management in Cambodia**

In the paediatric ward of a large refugee camp on the Thai–Cambodian border, traditional healers (Kru Khmer) were encouraged to work alongside health workers. Ward rounds included both clinical staff and Kru Khmer. Families liked this approach and the Kru Khmer provided valuable inputs to clinical decisions. Together, clinical staff and the Kru Khmer were able to provide complementary care, rather than competing treatment options. For example, a child might receive standard treatment for malaria along with a herbal potion or massage from a traditional healer. The Kru Khmer appreciated the recognition of their role and the health workers appreciated the cultural knowledge of the traditional healers.

Box 7.7 **Caregivers as peer role models**

One of the unexpected benefits of a drug efficacy trial in a refugee camp in the United Republic of Tanzania was the realization that those caring for under-fives enrolled in the trial were learning easier ways to give antimalarial drugs to the children. The caregivers would watch carefully when the team administered the drug used in the trial and ask questions about what they were doing. This provided an excellent opportunity to teach caregivers – mothers, fathers, older siblings and grandparents – safer techniques for holding the children while giving medications, different ways to give the drugs (e.g. crushing tablets to mix with liquid in a bottle or with a spoon), and what to do if a child vomited the drug shortly after administration. The caregivers said that, because regular health workers were often too busy to offer these explanations, they had not always known what to do with a child who refused to take medication or had vomited. Now that they knew what to do, they planned to share this knowledge with their family, friends and neighbours.

Box 7.8 **Involving the community in prevention in refugee camps on the Thai–Myanmar border**

Training community health educators
NGOs trained members of local ethnic minority groups as community health educators in refugee camps along the Thai–Myanmar border. During the mid-1990s, previously stable camp populations were forced to relocate because of shelling and border incursions. The community health educators ensured the continuity of malaria control activities: as the population moved to a new site, the educators were able to go from tent to tent and provide essential services including:

— information about the new location of health services and general health messages;
— active case detection for presumed cases of malaria and other common illnesses;
— education in the correct use of insecticide-treated nets.

Because they belonged to the same ethnic group as the displaced population, the community educators were able to bridge the gap between the refugees and the agencies working in malaria control. This was particularly important for some of the more isolated ethnic groups who had little previous exposure to or knowledge of this kind of health care.

Training community health workers
In the same camps, NGOs also trained community health workers to interpret the routine data that they were collecting, to increase their understanding of how this information could be used to design malaria control activities. This method, called community-oriented primary care, combined elements of primary health care, public health and community mobilization. Meetings and workshops were held on a regular basis to provide training for the community health workers and to review data collection and analysis, implementation, monitoring and evaluation of activities.

The example in Box 7.10 illustrates the importance of understanding the local context, showing how adapting symptom control measures to local belief systems can improve their acceptability.

Regular community meetings are important, to keep the community informed about malaria control activities, to provide them with an opportunity to raise concerns about malaria, and to find joint solutions to problems.

Box 7.9 **Community involvement in insecticide-treated materials programmes**

HealthNet International (HNI) has been actively involved in programmes to distribute insecticide-treated materials to Afghan refugees living in villages and resettlement camps in Pakistan (Hewitt et al., 1996; Rowland et al., 1996, 1999). Community involvement, and understanding of cultural practices, led to a creative adaptation. Instead of relying only on treated mosquito nets, HNI has also treated the traditional veils, or chadors, worn by women during the day and used by men and women as a top sheet at night. Treating chadors with permethrin was not only an effective protection measure but also culturally acceptable. This approach also provides protection to vulnerable groups that may not be able to afford to buy nets.

HNI also engaged community members in the re-treatment of nets. Village health workers, nominated by village committees, became responsible for re-treatment. This approach reduced operational costs and increased community participation in the ITN programme.[1]

[1] Rowland M. *Country presentations. Review of lessons learned: Afghanistan*. Oral presentation at the WHO Roll Back Malaria and Emergency and Humanitarian Action Expert Group Meeting on Malaria Control in Complex Emergencies, 1–2 December 1998.

Box 7.10 **Importance of understanding the local context**

Refugees from Angola have been settling in the north-west border area of Zambia since the late 1960s. Because both the displaced and host populations believe that people with fever should not drink water, promotion of hydration in people with febrile illness, particularly children, was failing. However, when food colouring and sugar were added to the water and the resulting solution was described as medicinal, hydration with this solution became acceptable.

Health education in malaria control
Establishing priorities

The goal of health education should be to inform populations at risk about behaviour changes that could reduce their risk of malaria infection and improve their management of malaria illness. Health education should specifically address the concerns identified by the displaced or refugee and host communities, in addition to the following issues:

— causes of malaria and the role of mosquitoes in transmission;
— the groups that are particularly vulnerable to malaria;
— the difference between uncomplicated and severe malaria;

— treatment of malaria;
— location and opening hours of health services;
— danger signs that mean a patient should go back to the clinic;
— measures that can be taken to protect against mosquito biting, including use of treated nets and other forms of personal protection.

The emphasis placed on these various issues will depend on the phase of the emergency. In the first few days of the acute phase it is essential that people know both how to recognize the signs of severe malaria and where and how to access treatment and care. As an emergency evolves and the situation stabilizes, more attention will be given to such issues as preventing transmission or sustaining preventive measures, for example by re-treating mosquito nets. The emphasis will also depend on the local context. For example, if the displaced population has moved from a non-malarious area to an area where malaria is a risk, health education about the risk of transmission will be important.

Designing health education

At the beginning of the acute phase of a complex emergency, when there are other more urgent priorities, it will not usually be possible to develop a "formal" health education programme. During this phase, information passed by word of mouth can be a useful way to publicize urgent messages in the community.

Once the situation stabilizes, a health education programme can be designed and implemented. It is important to invest time and resources in doing this with the community, who should be involved in designing and pretesting messages and in making any revisions necessary as a result of pretesting. Failing to do this can waste limited time and resources on producing ineffective messages and materials.

Health education should focus on learning (not teaching), active participation, action and behaviour change. The principles of successful health education include:

- *Defining the objectives of health education* – for example, the desired improvement in knowledge or change in behaviour, or how to build on existing knowledge, beliefs and behaviours.

- *Identifying the target audience* – for example, pregnant women, parents of young children, community leaders, traditional healers, drug sellers.

- *Defining the desired behaviours and developing clear messages* – in such a way that the target audience understands.

156

- *Providing information about what people can do* – for example where they can get nets or when to seek treatment – with a limited number of clear, simple messages, such as "Prompt treatment for fever saves lives", repeated in different ways.

- *Using methods that are culturally acceptable* – and appropriate for the target audience.

- *Delivering messages through trusted and respected individuals and channels.*

- *Providing training and materials* – to those who will conduct health education, for example, community educators, health workers, traditional healers.

Effective health communication depends, in part, on understanding aspects of the community that is being targeted with the message. Specific information from the targeted community, such as knowing where and how people expect to receive important information, will help to inform decisions about the design of your communication materials (see Box 7.11).

Implementing health education

In complex emergencies it is important to plan the timing of health education activities carefully.

- Avoid days when rations are being distributed or when cultural or religious events are taking place.

- Take advantage of occasions when people are already meeting together, for example meetings with block or camp leaders.

- Alert the community in advance about campaigns or activities, for example spraying or net re-treatment.

- Use opportunities to target specific groups, for example pregnant women and mothers of young children. In many emergency situations, women spend a lot of time waiting in outpatient clinics or at supplementary feeding centres; this time can be used for health education about some aspect of malaria, for example what to do when a child has fever. However, it is also important to address health education messages to men, as recent field experience indicates that, increasingly, men are also bringing sick children to clinics.

Box 7.11 **Communication channels, messages and methods**

Channels

Effective delivery of health education messages depends on choosing communication channels appropriate to the community's culture, knowledge, beliefs, values and literacy level. In some cultures, community leaders and elders may be the best people to transmit messages, while in others, teachers, health workers or the media may have more credibility. Messages can also be relayed through other types of community workers, such as those who dig latrines or do other manual tasks. Other possible channels for disseminating messages can include:

— camp management meetings
— health and water coordination meetings
— health facilities
— community health programmes, such as vaccination campaigns
— central message boards, particularly in transit areas.

Messages

The following principles should govern the development of messages:

■ Target the message to the lowest level of literacy.
■ Be clear about what people are expected to do and what the result of their action will be.
■ Ensure that messages are realistic and feasible.
■ Reflect local language and behaviours.
■ Ensure that messages are culturally acceptable.
■ Remember that messages will need to change as the situation changes.
■ Use creative approaches in the messages. For example, promoting ITNs may be more successful if the messages describe the nets as a way of "preventing nuisance insects from disturbing your sleep" as well as a way to prevent malaria.

Methods

The choice of methods must also be appropriate for the setting. Printed messages are fine for more literate populations, but oral and visual methods will be needed to convey messages to less literate populations. In most situations it is useful to use a mixture of methods. Possible methods include:

■ *Print* – posters, flipcharts and picture guides. These can combine words and pictures. Posters should be displayed in places where people will see them, e.g. clinics or registration centres. Flipcharts and picture guides are useful for teaching and health education sessions, e.g. about how to give an antimalarial drug to a young child.

■ *Oral* – talks, person-to-person communication, songs, poetry and informal conversations. Give talks to, for instance, religious or women's groups or at times when people are waiting, for instance at the clinic.

Box 7.11 *Continued*

- ■ *Visual* – drama, role-play and dance, or demonstrations. Drama and similar methods use stories to get across messages. Demonstrations are a useful way to show people how to do something, for example how to use a treated net.

- ■ *Media* – public broadcasting or radio. Megaphones or public announcements through loudspeakers are especially useful in the acute phase of an emergency when people are still arriving and residential blocks have not yet been established.

Monitoring and evaluation

As for other aspects of malaria control, community participation and health education activities must be monitored and evaluated. It is important to check whether or not these activities have succeeded in changing people's behaviour. For example, it may be necessary to assess whether there have been changes in use of individual protection methods – by monitoring and evaluating net coverage, proper net use, or re-treatment rates. Alternatively, it may be important to assess changes in treatment-seeking and case management – by monitoring and evaluating the number of children brought for treatment, treatment compliance, the length of time between initial symptoms and seeking care at a health care facility, or the number of return visits.

References

Bloland PB, Williams HA (2003). *Malaria control during mass population movements and natural disasters.* Roundtable on the demography of forced migration. Washington, DC, National Academies Press.

Hewitt SE et al. (1996). Self-protection from malaria vectors in Pakistan: an evaluation of popular existing methods and appropriate new techniques in Afghan refugee communities. *Annals of Tropical Medicine and Parasitology*, 90:337–344.

Médecins Sans Frontières (1997). *Refugee health. An approach to emergency situations.* London, Macmillan Educational.

Meek SR (1995). *Partnerships for change and communications: guidelines for malaria control.* Geneva, World Health Organization.

Person B, Cotton D (1996). A model of community mobilization for the prevention of HIV in women and infants. *Public Health Reports*, 3(Suppl. 1):89–98.

Rifkin S (1996). Rapid rural appraisal: its use and value for health planners and managers. *Public Administration*, 74:509–526.

Rowland M et al. (1996). Pyrethroid-impregnated bednets for personal protection against malaria for Afghan refugees. *Transactions of the Royal Society of Tropical Medicine and Hygiene*, 90:357–361.

Rowland M et al. (1999). Permethrin-treated chaddars and top-sheets: appropriate technology for protection against malaria in Afghanistan and other complex emergencies. *Transactions of the Royal Society of Tropical Medicine and Hygiene*, 93:465–472.

Watson T (1999). *Partnerships in the protection of refugees and other people at risk: emerging issues and work in progress.* Geneva, Office of the United Nations High Commissioner for Refugees, Centre for Documentation and Research (UNHCR Working Paper, No. 13).

Williams H (2001). Introduction. In: Williams H, ed. *Caring for those in crisis: integrating anthropology and public health in complex humanitarian emergencies.* Washington, DC, National Association for the Practice of Anthropology, American Anthropological Association (NAPA Bulletin 21):1–16.

Further reading

A tool box for building health communication capacity (1995). Washington DC, Academy for Educational Development.

Akua Agyepong I et al. (1995). *The malaria manual.* Geneva, World Health Organization (TDR/SER/MSR/95.1).

Bamberger M, ed. (2000). *Integrating quantitative and qualitative research in development projects.* Washington DC, World Bank.

Bernard H (1994). *Research methods in anthropology: qualitative and quantitative approaches*, 2nd ed. Thousand Oaks, CA, Sage Publications.

Brieger W (1996). Health education to promote community involvement in the control of tropical disease. *Acta Tropica*, 61:93–106.

Dawson S et al. (1993). *A manual for the use of focus groups.* Boston, MA, International Foundation for Developing Countries.

Debus M (1988). *Methodological review: a handbook for excellence in focus group research.* Washington, DC, Academy for Educational Development.

De Negri B et al. (1998). *Empowering communities: participatory techniques for community-based programme development.* Nairobi, Centre for African Family Studies.

Freudenberger K (1998). *Rapid rural appraisal (RRA) and participatory rural appraisal (PRA): a manual for CRS field workers and partners.* Baltimore, MD, Catholic Relief Services.

Geefhuysen C, Bennett E, Lewin N (1995). *Health information: its collection and use. A training manual for community workers.* Brisbane, University of Queensland Medical School.

Glanz K, Rimer B (1997). *Theory at a glance: a guide for health promotion practice.* Washington, DC, National Cancer Institute, US Department of Health and Human Services.

Scrimshaw N, Gleason G, eds (1992). *Rapid assessment procedures: qualitative methodologies for planning and evaluation of health related programmes.* Boston, MA, International Foundation for Developing Countries.

Squire C, Gerami N (1998). Afghan refugees in Iran: the needs of women and children. *Forced Migration Review*, 3:19–22.

Warren C (1988). *Gender issues in field research.* Thousand Oaks, CA, Sage Publications.

Weiss W, Bolton P (2000). *Training in qualitative research methods for PVOs and NGOs: a trainer's guide to strengthen program planning and evaluation.* Baltimore MD, Johns Hopkins University School of Public Health.

Weiss W, Bolton P, Shankar A (2000). *Rapid assessment procedures: a guide to understanding the perceived needs of refugees and internally displaced populations.* Baltimore MD, Johns Hopkins University School of Public Health (draft).

WHO (1996). *Malaria: a manual for community health workers.* Geneva, World Health Organization.

WHO (1997). *"Mucoore (trusted friend), let's share with others!"* Geneva, World Health Organization (TDR/GEN/97.1).

Williams H et al. (1999) A community perspective in the efficacy of malaria treatment options for children: Lundazi district, Zambia. *Tropical Medicine and International Health*, 10:641–652.

Winch P et al. (2000). *Qualitative research for improved health programs: a guide to manuals for qualitative and participatory research on child health, nutrition and reproductive health.* Baltimore MD, SARA/Johns Hopkins University School of Public Health.

CHAPTER 8

Operational research

This chapter:
- describes how malaria operational research can help to develop a more effective response in complex emergencies
- identifies priority areas for operational research
- outlines how to plan, design and implement operational research studies.

The essential interventions for malaria control in acute complex emergencies are increasingly well defined, with case management and the establishment of early warning systems for broader communicable diseases outbreaks as clear priorities. Beyond that, things are less certain and increasingly dependent on the local context – which is where operational research comes in.

By addressing practical issues, operational research guides the choice of the best interventions for the local context, and improves programme delivery and uptake by the target population. In its most straightforward form it provides the intelligence for simple programme troubleshooting.

Why malaria operational research is important in complex emergencies

There are many different approaches to malaria control and no approach is 100% effective or appropriate in every situation. The purpose of operational research is to improve control tools, their application and their impact.

There is growing recognition of the need for operational research in complex emergencies (see Boxes 8.1 and 8.2) and of the role that research can play in improving malaria control. Operational research can be used to identify locally effective treatments, appropriate prevention methods, and cultural and behavioural factors that contribute to the problem or limit the effectiveness of control measures. Because emergencies are fluid situations – moving from acute to chronic or post-conflict phases – the feasibility

---

Box 8.1 Types of operational research needed in complex emergencies

---

■ *Research that concerns locally specific issues* – which may need to be investigated in each and every emergency; for example, cultural beliefs about disease causation and health-seeking behaviour.

■ *Research that has general applicability to most emergencies* – which may require some input from specialists; for example, development research on insecticide-treated plastic sheeting and blankets.

The boundary between these two types of research is not always clear and emergency partners may often be involved in both. For example, after a new control or treatment intervention is developed it may need to be evaluated in emergency settings with different epidemiological and social conditions.

Box 8.2 Research roles of RBM in complex emergencies

■ Helping to establish operational research priorities and secure funding from potential donors.

■ Assisting donors by screening and endorsing operational research proposals.

■ Strengthening research skills of implementing agencies.

■ Providing direct technical support to agencies engaged in operational research in complex emergencies.

■ Publishing and sharing research findings through scientific and medical journals, web sites, newsletter updates and other media.

---

of approaches to malaria control may change as the situation progresses. Operational research can be used to identify the best approach in different phases of an emergency, and can help to guide necessary modifications as the situation changes. It can also help in assessing the effectiveness of case management and preventive measures or the impact of outbreak control. Integration of research with normal control activities has helped to solve malaria problems that have arisen in refugee camps in the complex emergencies in Afghanistan and Myanmar during the past two decades; examples are given in Chapters 5 and 6.

It is hoped that the examples provided and the issues identified in this chapter will encourage agencies working in emergencies to become involved in operational research, rather than to see it as the concern only of outside experts.

Guiding principles

In an emergency context, where resources are stretched and reduction of mortality is the priority, operational research must be:

— relevant and focused on priority local problems;
— kept as simple as possible;
— short term (3–6 months maximum), because of the risk that the situation will change before outcomes can be measured;
— designed to provide practical information to enable agencies to overcome acute operational problems and provide better control interventions;
— undertaken as far as possible by local staff, with external support if necessary, to build up local skills;
— planned and conducted with the involvement of the ministry of health (MOH) where feasible.

Strict criteria must be met before operational research is undertaken (see Box 8.3), and the results must be shared with government, NGOs and United Nations agencies with the aim of improving local malaria control practices and informing necessary policy changes.

The rights of individuals and communities to participate in surveys and studies must be protected and informed consent obtained. Approval from an ethics committee should be sought (see later in this chapter).

Priority research needs

In complex emergencies, the two most important areas of operational research are establishing the effectiveness of

— diagnosis and treatment
— prevention measures.

Other important areas include social and behavioural factors, strategies for delivery of preventive interventions, cost and cost-effectiveness of malaria control, and disease burden. Priority topics for operational research that have general applicability to most emergencies are summarized in Box 8.4.

Establishing accurate diagnosis and effective treatment

Operational research can help to assess the effectiveness of diagnosis and treatment. Prompt and accurate diagnosis is critical but often difficult in the acute phase of emergencies. The effectiveness of malaria treatment is affected by drug resistance and by issues related to treatment provision,

Box 8.3 **Criteria for operational research**

■ **Relevance**
How significant or severe is the problem?
Can it be solved by other means that do not require research?

■ **Avoid duplication**
Has the research already been done somewhere else?
Was the context comparable?

■ **Feasibility**
How adequate are security, expertise, staff, time, and budget?

■ **Political acceptability**
Does the research have the interest and support of the MOH, UN agencies and NGO partners?

■ **Applicability**
Will the findings be applied and necessary resources be made available?

■ **Cost-effectiveness**
Will the time, money and human resources invested justify the expected result?
What difference will the study make to existing programmes?

■ **Timeliness**
Will the findings be available in time to inform decision-making?

■ **Ethics**
Is the research methodology ethical?
Can informed consent be obtained?
When should the study end and its findings be put into practice?

such as access to facilities, treatment-seeking behaviour and adherence to treatment, quality of drugs and quality of care.

Rapid diagnostic tests

Clinical diagnosis of malaria is inaccurate and unreliable while laboratory confirmation using microscopy is not always feasible in complex emergencies. Rapid diagnostic tests (RDTs) have many potential advantages in emergency situations. They are likely to be most useful during the acute phase for monitoring the accuracy of clinical diagnosis and rapidly assessing malaria prevalence, and as an interim diagnostic tool before the establishment of microscopy. However, research is needed to answer questions about the use of RDTs in complex emergencies, including:

• Does the use of RDTs improve treatment-seeking behaviour or alter patient adherence to treatment?

Box 8.4 **Priority research areas with general applicability**

Insecticide-treated blankets
There is scientific evidence for the effectiveness against malaria of in situ treatment of blankets/bedsheets with permethrin in camp and village settings. Research in Asia, and to a lesser extent in Africa, suggests that permethrin-treated blankets and sheets could play an important role in individual protection (Rowland et al., 1999). Priorities for research include assessing their suitability in different cultures and climatic conditions, their efficacy under highly endemic conditions, especially in Africa, long-lasting treatment processes and formulations, and the suitability of different blanket materials. Operational constraints (mass dipping/spraying of blankets) currently limit their use in emergencies. The duration of effectiveness of pretreated blankets (either stockpiled or in field use) still needs to be evaluated.

Insecticide-treated plastic sheeting (ITPS)
Treated canvas tents have been shown to provide protection (Bouma et al., 1996), but most agencies are moving towards provision of plastic sheeting rather than tents. ITPS impregnated with deltamethrin or permethrin during manufacture has been shown to kill mosquitoes in small-scale field trials in Pakistan (Graham et al., 2002), and community trials are underway in west Africa. In situations where ITPS that is already commercially available is being used, its efficacy (and duration of efficacy) against malaria and its safety under field conditions must be monitored and reported to build up the evidence base.

Burden of disease in complex emergencies
Better information is needed about the contribution of emergencies to the global malaria disease burden.

- Would use of RDTs change outcomes, such as morbidity and mortality?
- What is the cost-effectiveness of RDTs compared with other methods of diagnosis?

Drug resistance

Artemisinin-based combination therapy (ACT) must be used as first-line treatment for falciparum malaria for all populations living in complex emergencies. Its efficacy depends on resistance to the artemisinin-partner drug. When choosing a new ACT as local drug policy, it should have at least 95% efficacy. In chronic-phase emergencies, 2-yearly therapeutic efficacy testing in sentinel sites should be carried out to ascertain that the efficacy of the ACT remains above 90%. Where treatment failure is common, it is important to find out whether there might a resistance problem (see Box 8.5). Information about drug resistance in countries is available on the WHO RBM web site (http://www.who.int/malaria/resistance.html). Also on this web site is the current protocol for assessing in vivo drug response (see also Chapter 5). The standardized in vivo test includes both clinical and parasitological response, and is:

— applicable to all epidemiological conditions;
— feasible in emergency situations where there is adequate microscopy and cases can be followed up;
— suitable for evaluating treatment efficacy in areas of intense malaria transmission and, if follow-up is extended, for evaluating the efficacy of drugs with a longer half-life, such as mefloquine, in areas of unstable malaria transmission.

For the following reasons, in vivo testing has some limitations in emergency situations:

— patients need to be followed up for 14 days or longer;
— tracing of defaulters may be difficult.

Treatment provision

Operational research can identify both the factors that prevent people from receiving effective malaria treatment and what needs to be done to improve the quality of treatment. For example, it can help to improve access to treatment by finding out whether health facilities are easily accessible and located in appropriate sites, and whether different cultural and ethnic groups have equal access to treatment. It can reveal much about treatment-seeking behaviour and, for example, whether all sections of the population are using health facilities and, if not, why not.

Box 8.5 **Identifying drug resistance in Afghan refugee camps**

Outpatient records in one Afghan refugee camp in Pakistan showed that 50% of falciparum cases were re-attending within 1–4 weeks of initial treatment. This suggested two possible problems – resistance to chloroquine or poor patient adherence. An in vivo survey was conducted and the results showed resistance frequency to be 62% (Shah et al., 1997). In vivo surveys carried out subsequently in refugee camps in other parts of Pakistan found that the frequency of resistance varied little and was no different from the frequencies found in the Pakistani population (Rowland et al., 1997b).

Operational research can also be used to monitor standards of care, to ensure that the quality of treatment provided by MOH, NGO and private health facilities is adequate and that health workers adhere to recommended drug treatment protocols. Regular surveys of public- and private-sector coverage and prescription practices are recommended in every phase of an emergency. Such research, if followed up by training and accreditation of competent practitioners, can help to improve standards, enable the population to make informed choices about health providers, and assist the MOH to regulate or maintain standards in both public and private sectors.

Drug quality
Counterfeit artemisinin derivatives are increasingly common because of the high monetary value of ACT. Trademarks are easily forged and it can be dangerous to buy drugs in the market place or from other than official sources. The quality of ACT treatment can be assured by obtaining supplies only from reputable pharmaceutical companies/agencies – and preferably directly from producers. Where there are doubts, operational research is important to assure drug quality. Generic drugs, if used, should be properly assayed since they often vary in quality. Some locally produced antimalarials may contain insufficient active ingredient for effective treatment, which may result in patient deaths.

Establishing effective prevention
Operational research can help to assess the effectiveness of prevention measures. It can play an important role in evaluating the effectiveness of different transmission control and individual protection measures and of component elements of these measures, such as community education, behaviour, and intervention delivery methods.

Indoor residual spraying
Indoor residual spraying (IRS) of insecticide is a commonly used method of community vector control in emergencies. It requires coverage of ≥ 85% of dwellings to be fully effective and is generally not feasible during acute emergencies, except possibly in well-organized transit camp settings (see Chapter 6). In IRS programmes that continue for more than one spraying cycle, operational research is required to monitor the effectiveness and residual life of sprayed insecticide. This is most easily accomplished by periodic WHO cone bioassay tests (see Annex VI). Operational research has helped to formulate guiding principles on IRS (see Box 8.6) but more

Box 8.6 **Lessons learned from research into IRS in Afghan refugee camps**[1]

■ IRS in Afghan refugee camps is most effective if campaigns are undertaken at/before the beginning of the transmission season.
■ Procurement and application are often too slow to control outbreaks when the transmission period is short or seasonal.
■ Pyrethroid insecticides should be used – they are safer to handle, lighter to transport, and never less effective than organophosphates or carbamates.
■ IRS should become more focused after the acute phase, and targeted at areas selected on the basis of epidemiological indicators.
■ IRS is more effective than ITNs when applied for just one or two seasons.

These lessons may guide thinking in other settings but are likely to need adaptation and possibly additional research for different environments.

[1] Rowland, 1999; Rowland et al., 1997a.

research is needed to answer general questions, covering aspects that include the following:

— comparison with the cost-effectiveness of alternative control measures, because IRS is expensive and may not be financially sustainable year after year in chronic emergency situations (Kolaczinski et al., 2004);

— comparative trials of pyrethroids and organophosphates or carbamates in areas where pyrethroid resistance is emerging, as in *A. gambiae* in west Africa (Chandre et al., 1999) and in *A. funestus* in southern Africa (Hargreaves et al., 2000).

A successful IRS campaign requires good organization and can easily fail to produce the desired result unless well planned and monitored. Campaign timing in relation to transmission season is an important indicator. Monitoring of programme quality should take place during the IRS application (indicators a–d below) and 1 month afterwards (indicator e):

a) Coverage = number of dwellings sprayed/number of dwellings in targeted area (%).

b) Insecticide used per dwelling = quantity of insecticide use/number of dwellings sprayed (a measure of efficiency and correct use of insecticide).

c) User acceptability pre-spray = % of households refusing to be sprayed.

d) % of spray pumps properly maintained and still working during and at the end of the campaign.

e) User acceptability post-spray = % of dwellings replastered or washed, or % of householders complaining about IRS.

Additional indicators for research are the impact of IRS on malaria incidence rates or prevalence; reductions in vector density; and insecticide quality and residual life on sprayed surfaces. (The last two require an entomologist.)

Insecticide treatment of domestic animals

Insecticide treatment of domestic animals has been shown in trials in refugee camps to be a very cheap and effective method of malaria control in areas where people keep livestock and vectors feed primarily on animals (Rowland et al., 2001). This method could substitute for indoor residual spraying in south Asia and the Middle East where vectors feed mainly on animals. In particular, it has the potential to control malaria in emergencies in Afghanistan and Tajikistan. Operational research is needed to evaluate its potential role and feasibility in emergencies.

Insecticide-treated nets

Insecticide-treated nets (ITNs) have been shown to provide protection in many settings (see Chapter 6) and are effective as a community control measure if population coverage in excess of 60% (some studies indicate 50%) is achieved. At lower coverage rates, ITNs provide protection for each person sleeping under a net. Although ITNs are considered appropriate for epidemic or outbreak control only under very specific conditions (Nájera, 1996), and their use in acute emergencies is limited mainly to personal protection for priority vulnerable groups, there is increasing evidence of the effectiveness of ITNs in the post-acute phase of emergencies (Rowland et al., 2002; Kolaczinski et al., 2004).

ITNs work well in Africa against all malaria vector species *if used regularly and correctly*, but they are not effective in every epidemiological context. Among Karen refugees on the Thai–Myanmar border, for example, sleeping under treated nets provided limited protection because the local vector bites early in the evening, before people go to bed (Luxemburger et al., 1994). Operational research is therefore needed on vector biting cycles and on the disease impact of treated nets in regions where effectiveness is currently unknown.

ITNs may not be the best solution in the acute phase of emergencies. Community distribution to vulnerable groups should be considered only if ITNs have been stockpiled in advance, the community is in the habit of using them, and no community vector control interventions (IRS) are ongoing. Before ITN coverage is expanded, basic research is needed to:

— find out the previous experience of nets among the displaced populations, whether they want or would use nets, and the importance of nets relative to other priorities;
— develop appropriate information materials and evaluate instructions on net use and care;
— find out about appropriate sizes and shapes for nets;
— find out what people do with the nets they are given, whether nets are used, who uses them, and what proportion is resold;
— monitor the frequency of net washing.

Programme monitoring for ITN programmes should take place at distribution (indicator a below), and at 1 month (indicators b and c) and 6 months (indicator d) after the intervention:

a) Coverage = number of ITNs distributed / target population size (%).
b) Utilization rate = number of people using ITN/number of people given ITNs (%).
c) Retention rate = number of people retaining ITNs/number of people originally given ITNs (%).
d) Deterioration rate = average number of holes per ITN.

   Note: Even nets with some holes can be protective against mosquitoes if they are treated with pyrethroid insecticide – this is one of the purposes of the insecticide treatment.

Operational research can provide important insights into issues of broader applicability, such as the impact of free distribution of ITNs on the private sector and on future willingness to buy nets, and the effectiveness of insecticide treatments of nets (see Annex VI).

Alternative individual protection and community control approaches

Insecticide-treated nets are an expensive investment to make if their acceptability or effectiveness is uncertain, and they may not be practical when populations are living in tents or under plastic sheeting. Further operational research is needed to assess the potential of alternative approaches, such as pyrethroid treatment of top-sheets, blankets, tents or the plastic tarpaulins that are increasingly being used as an alternative to tents by UNHCR (see Chapter 6). One potential advantage of these materials is that they are already being distributed in acute emergencies; if they could be rendered protective against malaria there would be a dual benefit with no extra demands being placed on logistics. Research in Asia indicates that insecticide-treated plastic sheeting (ITPS) may, like IRS, provide community protection through mass killing effect of the mosquito population – but no personal protection from mosquito bites.

Further research is required to assess:

— the potential of treated top-sheets and blankets in different cultural, epidemiological and climatic settings in Africa, to determine the most suitable blanket materials for treatment and different methods of treatment (e.g. spraying or immersion);
— the potential of ITPS, which is impregnated during manufacture and currently being pilot-tested in west Africa.

Protection from malaria in pregnancy

Strategies to protect pregnant women are described in Chapters 5 and 6. Research is needed to identify the best ways to target ITN programmes at pregnant women, and to evaluate the effectiveness of intermittent preventive treatment (IPT) with sulfadoxine–pyrimethamine (SP) delivered as a part of antenatal care in complex emergencies. Information on the effectiveness of IPT (measured as prevention of severe anaemia and low birth weight) in areas where it is being implemented is also needed to inform the continuing broader debate about use of IPT in areas with relatively high levels of SP resistance (see Chapter 5).

Understanding social and behavioural factors

Successful malaria control depends on agencies understanding communities and communities understanding and using prevention and treatment measures. It is crucial to understand what people know, believe and do about malaria. Social and behavioural research is important for designing effective interventions and can shed light on why a particular intervention fails to be accepted (see Box 8.7).

Operational research on the following social and behavioural issues could strengthen planning and implementation. Chapter 7 and Annex VII provide additional ideas for questions that may need to be asked.

Treatment-seeking and access to care

- What local terms do people use to describe febrile illness?
- What perceptions do people have about the causes of febrile illness?
- What influences treatment-seeking?

Box 8.7 **Understanding social and behavioural factors**

KAP survey in eastern Democratic Republic of the Congo
In eastern Democratic Republic of the Congo, health data showed that only 20–30% of the population were using health services. A knowledge, attitudes and practices (KAP) survey was conducted by Merlin into treatment-seeking practices in the community, barriers to accessing health care, and knowledge and beliefs about malaria. The findings showed that the main barrier to accessing health care was economic, because of the cost-recovery system in place.

Sociobehavioural research in Zambia
In Zambia, behavioural research showed that families were not bringing children with severe malaria for treatment because they believed that the cause was spiritual and that the disease therefore needed to be treated by a traditional healer.

- Where is treatment obtained? Health services, traditional healers, private practitioners?
- When is treatment sought? Is there a delay? How long before treatment is sought from a clinic?
- What access do people have to antimalarials? Does the private sector provide effective drugs? How is the supply of drugs regulated or maintained? Do traditional healers prescribe antimalarials?
- Does the population accept the recommended standard treatment for malaria? Is camp treatment policy different from their former experience of treatment?
- How do people feel about antimalarial safety and efficacy?
- What are the barriers to treatment and care? Are services accessible?
- What role is played by intermediaries, such as other family members, in accessing care?
- Does security affect access to care?
- Are some groups excluded on grounds of sex or ethnic origin?

Prevention
- What individual protection measures were traditionally used?
- What measures are currently acceptable?
- What is the market value of materials treated with insecticide? Is reselling or an illegal market likely to undermine the effectiveness of these materials?
- What items do people most value? Are nets valued or are they sold?
- Does the displaced population have employment and income?

- Who makes household expenditure decisions?
- Who should be targeted with health information?

Operational research can provide information on people's beliefs and knowledge about prevention, and useful insight for ITN programmes on family sleeping arrangements, sex or age differences in net use, net washing practices, and the proportion of the population using distributed nets.

Social information can be collected by interviewing community leaders or by conducting participatory community research (see Chapter 7), sometimes also called Rapid Participatory Appraisal or Rapid Ethnographic Assessment.

Identifying sustainable strategies to deliver preventive interventions

It is now generally accepted that malaria services must be free of charge to users in complex emergencies. During the acute – and to a lesser extent the chronic – phase of complex emergencies, most agencies do indeed provide preventive interventions such as nets and insecticide treatment, free of charge to the affected population. However, as an emergency situation resolves, RBM partners need to consider how to move to sustainable delivery of preventive interventions, including cost recovery. This can be difficult when the affected population has become used to receiving services free of charge.

Various strategies have been used including, for example, social marketing and private-sector provision of nets and insecticide. Operational research is needed to identify the strategies that are most appropriate and to answer questions about:

- *Accessibility*
  Which delivery strategies are cost-effective and achieve best coverage and uptake?

- *Affordability*
  What are people willing and able to pay?
  What is the socioeconomic status of buyers and non-buyers, and how can this information be used to support more effective promotion?
  How can the most vulnerable be identified and protected?
  Is there is a need for subsidies or credit schemes?
  What is the best coverage achievable when nets are sold, and is this good enough to control malaria in the community?

- *Demand creation*
  What is the best way to get the message across?
  What methods work best in emergencies – mass media or person-to-person?

- *Monitoring*
  How can behaviour change and correct use best be monitored?

- *Insecticide re-treatment*
  What can be done to encourage people to retreat their nets?

Understanding the economics of malaria control

The costs and cost-effectiveness of malaria control in the acute phase of complex emergencies are still poorly documented. This is an area where more research is needed, especially in relation to the burden of malaria disease in emergencies (see below) and cases and mortality averted by different control interventions. Economic analysis of malaria control in emergencies should be feasible, because many agencies maintain detailed expenditure records for financial reporting to donors.

More is known about the post-emergency economics of malaria control. For example, studies have compared the cost-effectiveness of IRS and ITNs in Africa and Asia (Curtis et al., 1999; Rowland, 1999). More research is needed to identify prevention and treatment approaches that will be financially sustainable after the withdrawal of donor funding.

Understanding the burden of disease in complex emergencies

Current estimates of the contribution of malaria in complex emergencies to the global malaria burden are rough, as they are based on country population data and assume uniform mortality across highly endemic areas in Africa, irrespective of local social conditions. Studies of the burden of malaria disease at different stages of complex emergencies are needed – information for various emergency settings would give insight into the true contribution of complex emergencies to the global malaria burden.

As discussed in Chapter 2, cross-sectional surveys should form part of initial assessment and should be repeated at regular intervals as and when operational, social, and epidemiological conditions change, since changing situations will require different interventions. Surveillance (see Chapter 3) is a further operational research tool – without accurate surveillance it is impossible to make informed judgements about progress.

Measuring the effectiveness of outbreak control

Surveillance can also be used as an operational research tool to evaluate the impact of outbreak control interventions (see Chapters 3 and 4). In Afghan refugee camps, for example, it was suspected that IRS with the insecticide malathion was no longer working very effectively. In a pilot study carried out the following year, six refugee camps were sprayed with malathion as usual and a further six camps were sprayed with the pyrethroid lambda-cyhalothrin. Cross-sectional prevalence surveys before and after spraying confirmed that lambdacyhalothrin was giving better control than malathion, and policy was changed (Rowland, Hewitt & Durrani, 1994). Other indicators that might be used for measuring control impact, depending on the resources available, include the number of clinical malaria cases presenting at clinics, spleen rates in children, prevalence of anaemia, and mosquito population density.

Understanding post-emergency restratification of malaria

Emergency situations can affect the pattern of malaria in a country. As discussed earlier in this handbook, *P. falciparum* has re-emerged in Afghanistan and Tajikistan as a direct result of population movement during conflict (Pitt et al., 1998; Rowland et al., 2002a). Other consequences of emergencies – changes in land use and agriculture, breakdown in irrigation systems, migration to cities and increased urbanization – can also affect the pattern of malaria. Research is important to identify these changes.

Research using appropriate tools – sero-epidemiological surveys of malaria exposure, cross-sectional parasite prevalence surveys, Geographic Information Systems and remote sensing of land use – can help to restratify malaria epidemiology and ensure that control resources are targeted effectively.

Operational research procedures
Research planning

Malaria operational research and malaria control programmes are similar in terms of the process of planning and design, the tools and indicators used, and the approaches used for monitoring and evaluation. However, operational research differs from control programmes in that it starts from a position of uncertainty, or lack of knowledge, and aims to identify the best solution – which may involve comparing the results of a number of approaches.

The steps in developing an operational research plan (see Table 8.1) are the same whether the aim is to improve an existing programme or to de-

Table 8.1 **Steps in developing an operational research plan**

Questions	Steps	Important elements
What is the problem?	Statement and definition	
What information is already available?	Review published literature, government or agency records	Scientific, medical and "grey" literature
What is the purpose?	Formulate objectives	Research questions or hypotheses
What additional information or data are needed? How should information/data be collected?	Develop research methodology	Type of study; data collection techniques; variables; sampling; data collection plan; analysis plan; ethical considerations; pilot study or pretest
How will the results be used?	Plan for use and dissemination of results	Involve future beneficiaries in planning or execution of research
Who will do what and when?	Develop work plan	Personnel scheduling; monitoring; evaluation
What is needed?	Plan resources and budget	Staff; equipment; material support; finance
How should the argument be presented to authorities, partners, donors?	Develop proposal	

velop a new approach to malaria control. Important aspects of the design of operational research include:

— agreeing clear objectives;
— setting realistic targets;
— anticipating outcomes;
— planning activities according to a strict timeframe;
— establishing a system for monitoring – with appropriate technical and process indicators to measure progress – and evaluation.

Good organization and planning are vital: if an activity is not carried out properly or an output is not recorded properly, the results may be unclear and interpretation of the findings will be difficult.

It is particularly important to plan at the design stage how data will be collected and analysed. Planning data collection helps to clarify activities (quality control checks, sorting and processing, analysis), minimize errors, avoid unnecessary delays, and organize human and material resources. Planning how data will be analysed helps to formulate clear and specific objectives and determine what information should be collected in the first place.

A pretest of a particular research component or a pilot study of the entire research procedure with a small sample may help to identify potential problems, allowing necessary revisions to be made before research is implemented on a larger scale.

Deciding on the type of operational research
Study design
There are three types of study design:

— descriptive
— analytical
— experimental.

Descriptive studies
A descriptive study is the systematic collection and presentation of data to describe a particular situation. Examples of descriptive studies include an initial assessment of malaria in an emergency, a baseline malaria prevalence survey, and a survey of how many families own mosquito nets. Descriptive studies can be qualitative or quantitative.

- *Qualitative research* – may be concerned with attitudes or opinions that may change over time, or characteristics of particular groups; it usually focuses on small samples to allow variables to be explored in depth.

- *Quantitative research* – usually covers a larger population, but can involve qualitative research on a smaller sub-sample. For example, estimating the extent of net ownership in a population would require several hundred respondents to be surveyed, but discovering the reasons for owning or not owning a net would require in-depth interviews with a randomly selected sub-sample of owners and non-owners.

Analytical studies
Analytical studies try to establish causes or risk factors for malaria in a more rigorous way than descriptive studies; they include case–control studies (see Box 8.8) and cohort studies.

- In a *case–control study*, one group with the disease (cases) is compared with another without the disease (controls), to look for differences be-

Box 8.8 **Case–control study of the impact of ITNs in a complex emergency in Afghanistan**[1]

The impact and coverage of distribution of insecticide treated nets (ITNs) can be estimated using routine data collected by passive case detection at field clinics. Data from the microscopy registers of Behsud clinic in eastern Afghanistan were as follows:

Blood smears	Falciparum-positive (cases)	Falciparum-negative (controls)	Total
ITN user	52 (a)	610 (b)	662 (e)
Non-user	439 (c)	1958 (d)	2397 (f)
Total			3059 (g)

These data were used to estimate individual effectiveness through a case–control study. Slides that were positive for *P. falciparum* were considered to be cases, and slides that were negative were considered to be controls. Using the data collected, the odds ratio (ad/bc) = 0.38, so individual protective effectiveness = 1 – odds ratio = 0.62 or 62% (confidence interval 48–72%).

The data were also used to estimate **the proportion of the population covered with ITNs** (e/g) = 0.22.

The impact on malaria morbidity in the population, or **community effectiveness** = individual effectiveness x coverage, which in this community is 0.62 x 0.22 = 14%. It was therefore concluded that 14% (confidence interval 11–16%) of the total malaria cases in the community were prevented by the ITN distribution programme.

[1] Rowland et al., 2002b.

tween them – for example, in ITN use, housing, proximity to breeding sites – that might explain the difference in disease rates. Case–control studies are cheap and quick, and are therefore the method of choice for measuring the impact of an intervention in emergency conditions. Such studies are informative, provided that cases and controls are well matched.

- In a *cohort study*, a group exposed to a risk factor (the study group) is compared with a group that is not exposed (control group) over the same period of time. Both groups are selected at the same time and followed up for an equal period of time.

Cohort studies take longer than case–control studies and are usually labour-intensive and are more expensive. In emergency situations it can be difficult to identify all cases and to ensure follow-up over time because of population movement. For these reasons, cohort studies are more appropriate for stable, long-term refugee camps.

Experimental studies

An experimental study is a type of cohort study in which units are randomly allocated to an intervention (expected to reduce the risk of malaria) while other units are not. The intervention effect is measured by comparing the risk of malaria between the two groups. The randomized units might be individuals (for example, in a drug trial), families (for example, in a treated net protection trial) or communities (for example, in comparing indoor spraying campaigns of villages).

The unit of allocation may be a group if:

— the intervention is to be applied on a community-wide basis, such as many educational interventions;
— it is logistically easier to administer the intervention to groups than to individuals;
— the purpose is to reduce transmission of malaria in an area;
— delivery systems for the intervention are being tested or compared.

A double-blind randomized controlled trial is the "gold standard" for assessing efficacy because any intervention effect will be unambiguous. Units are allocated randomly to eliminate potential bias due to unforeseen factors. The double-blind approach, in which neither the researcher not the participant is aware of who is allocated to the intervention group or who to the control group, eliminates potential bias in the assessment of impact of an intervention. Deciding what the control group receives can involve difficult ethical issues, and these are discussed in more detail below.

Sampling and study size

A representative sample should possess all the characteristics of the population from which it is drawn. Approaches to sampling include:

- *Simple random sampling.* Each unit in the sampling frame has an equal chance of being selected. It may be difficult to take a simple random sample because of logistics or problems of excluding neighbours. In systematic sampling, units are taken at regular intervals. Stratified sampling selects representative subgroups or strata (for example, age or ethnic groups) in proportion to the population structure.

- *Cluster sampling.* A random sample of villages or camps is chosen, from which all individuals within the particular section of the population being studied (e.g. children under 5 years of age) are selected for the intervention. Cluster sampling is logistically easier, but more likely to be unrepresentative, although the risk of this can be reduced if the number of clusters is 20 or more.

Study size is important. If the study is too small it may fail to detect important effects or estimate effects too inaccurately; if it is too large it will use more resources than necessary. The study size should have adequate power (typically, at least 80% chance) to detect an effect large enough to be of practical importance, especially when the impact of new interventions is being evaluated. Computer programmes, such as EpiInfo, can be used to calculate required sample sizes.

Losses to follow-up are likely in refugee or displaced populations or in chronic emergency conditions. For example, during a 1-year study of insecticide-treated top-sheets in Kabul, Afghanistan, more than 30% of the study population moved house because of security problems. In emergency situations the sample size may need to be increased to allow for such higher losses to follow-up. For example, if sample size calculations indicate that 560 subjects are required and a 30% loss is predicted, the sample size should be increased to 800. The higher the rate of loss to follow-up, the less reliable the study results will be, particularly if it affects case and control groups unequally.

Other factors that determine the size of a study include availability of staff, transport, laboratory capacity, time and money.

Ethical considerations

Ethical considerations are particularly important in studies of refugee and displaced populations and the following issues are critical:

- Any research protocol that involves people should pass formal review by an ethical committee.

- Research should follow the guiding principles for research in the *Helsinki Declaration* of 1964, which is available at http://onlineethics.org/reseth/helsinki.html). These principles are further elaborated with respect to developing countries in the *International ethical guidelines for biomedical research involving human subjects* (CIOMS, 2002).

- Research for populations affected by complex emergencies is essential, but these vulnerable and socially and economically deprived groups must not be used in research that will mainly benefit more privileged groups.

181

- Informed consent must be obtained from all participants; it is the investigator's responsibility to ensure that subjects are fully informed of the potential risks and benefits of participating in a study.

- Intervention trials on refugees should be undertaken only when there is uncertainty about the potential benefit. If a previous study provides evidence for a benefit there is no justification for a trial unless there is good reason to believe that the results might be different in the present population or locality.

Choice of "control" interventions is a difficult ethical issue. The accepted principle is that any new intervention should be compared with the best intervention currently available. Comparison with a placebo or "no intervention" control group is acceptable only if no other effective intervention is known or if a known intervention is too expensive for general application. It is important to take account of the following:

- If an intervention is already being used, its withdrawal for the purposes of a research study would be unethical.

- If it is not clear whether an intervention already in use is still efficacious, a randomized trial comparing a promising new treatment with the existing treatment would be justified.

- If there are insufficient resources to meet the needs of everyone (which is usually the case), distribution might be randomized to enable an unequivocal assessment to be made (see Example 1 in Box 8.9).

- It is acceptable to try a new intervention that might be equivalent, or even slightly inferior, to another if it is cheaper, easier to implement, more sustainable, associated with fewer adverse reactions, or more acceptable to the community than the existing intervention. This situation may arise after a conflict when there is a need to develop interventions that can be sustained with limited resources by the national public health system.

Some agencies may prefer to conduct a comparative trial (see Example 2 in Box 8.9) rather than a randomized controlled trial, as there is no risk of withholding a beneficial treatment.

Community involvement

Active community cooperation is essential in most operational research studies. It is important to involve community leaders in research planning and design from the start. Depending on the type of study, participation

Box 8.9 **Different approaches to researching new interventions in Pakistan**

Example 1

When insecticide-treated nets were first introduced in Pakistan it was unclear whether they would prevent malaria since there was no tradition of using nets. The few nets made available by donors were given to randomly selected families in the camp rather than to a single cluster of families, and a similarly randomly selected group of families served as a control. After 6 months, when a preventive effect had been demonstrated and NGOs and donors were confident that the nets would make an impact, nets were made available to other families (Rowland et al., 1996).

Example 2

National policy in Pakistan included spraying with the insecticide malathion, against malaria. UNHCR felt committed to spraying with malathion in Afghan refugee camps in Pakistan, even though there was little evidence that it made any difference to malaria incidence. To evaluate a new candidate insecticide, it was decided that it would be more ethical to randomizing camps to be sprayed with either malathion or the new insecticide than to withdraw malathion altogether and compare camps sprayed with the new insecticide against camps that were not sprayed at all (Rowland et al., 1994).

may be passive – such as consenting to house spraying or disease monitoring, or active – such as using ITNs or other behaviour-change interventions.

Outcome measures

The most commonly used outcome measures in malaria operational research are:

— disease incidence
— disease prevalence
— intermediate variables, such as vector density or human behaviour change.

In studies of malaria control interventions in emergency situations, the difference in incidence or prevalence of disease in the intervention and control groups is the most relevant outcome. Once a disease surveillance and monitoring system is in place (see Box 8.10), it is simpler and more definitive to measure changes in disease outcome than to attempt to measure intermediate effects (such as changes in vector-biting density, or in knowledge, attitudes and behaviour). However, understanding intermediate variables is useful for refining or improving an intervention or explaining how it works.

Box 8.10 **Organizing laboratory support for research trials**

Microscopy is the most reliable method of detecting malaria parasites and provides the "gold standard" for assessing research trial outcome. The organization of a laboratory to support a research trial in the field differs from that of a standard laboratory for clinical diagnosis, because the objective in a trial or in surveillance surveys is to process large numbers of samples. In particular:

■ Quality control procedures are essential because of the repetitive nature of the work.
■ Random samples of slides should be re-examined at an external reference laboratory.
■ The re-examination should be blind to the original results and should focus on negative smears, asexual parasite counts, and correct identification of malaria species.

Where the intermediate variables are technical or require specialized advice, help should be sought from international or local experts.

The most useful method for monitoring malaria infection (see also Chapters 2 and 3) is a cross-sectional parasite prevalence survey, which:

— can be done even when health facilities are very basic;
— requires microscopy or rapid testing to determine parasite rates – supported by data on fever rates, temperature, packed cell volume, spleen rates and anaemia;
— will identify most infections and allow estimation of incidence rate, if conducted every 2 weeks.

If clinics are well established and well used – for example, when services are provided free of charge – passive case detection can provide good proxy estimates of incidence rate, provided that the size of the catchment population is known.

Although entomological surveys are important in initial assessment of a potential malaria problem and in identifying control solutions, they require technical expertise that may not be available to many agencies working in emergency situations. Assistance can be obtained from WHO.

Using study results
Dissemination of findings
Whether the results of research are positive or negative, they must be reported to national health officials in the MOH, to donor agencies, community leaders and participants, and to appropriate health and scientific

journals. The findings and any implications for policy should be discussed with the MOH and with disease control authorities such as WHO, UNHCR and leading NGOs.

Moving from operational research to programme development

Using research findings to guide programme development is critical. Successful new interventions may have to be integrated into current control programmes, and strategies to do this may need to be developed. The case studies below – one on treatment of drug-resistant malaria in Thailand and the other on prevention of malaria in Afghanistan – illustrate how simple, practical and relevant operational research can contribute to more efficient and effective malaria control programmes.

Case Study 1. Treatment research (Nosten et al., 2000)

Background

In Karen refugee camps on the western border of Thailand, *P. falciparum* had become resistant to most of the available antimalarial drugs.

Methods, results and lessons learned

The in vivo response of falciparum malaria to drug treatment has been monitored in the camps since 1985, when diagnostic and treatment facilities were first set up:

- Access to effective antimalarials was strictly controlled, and treatment given only after microscopic confirmation of malaria, to ensure accurate records and reliable estimates of incidence rate.
- In in vivo surveys, cases were monitored weekly to estimate the clinical and parasitological efficacy of the drug regimens.

This research programme of resistance monitoring and clinical epidemiology resulted in a drug treatment policy that stopped the spread of resistance. Using an artesunate–mefloquine regimen, patient cure rates have remained stable at over 95% for the past several years, while incidence rates in the catchment population have fallen by more than two-thirds over the same period. The methods used, main results and impact are summarized in the following table.

Dates	Observation	New treatment response	Interpretation and effects
Before 1984	Failure of chloroquine and then of sulfadoxine–pyrimethamine (SP) to cure falciparum malaria due to selection of drug-resistant strains	Introduction of mefloquine (15 mg/kg), initially combined with SP (MSP) in late 1984	Mefloquine overcomes resistance to chloroquine and SP and restores the cure rate to 98%
1985–90	Cure rates decline over the next 4 years despite strict control of drug use; incidence of falciparum malaria rises	MSP replaced by high-dose mefloquine (25 mg/kg)	Mefloquine resistance developing, leading to increased rates of transmission; high-dose mefloquine restores efficacy temporarily
1991–94	Failure rates with high-dose mefloquine rise inexorably, accompanied by higher gametocyte carriage	Artesunate and high-dose mefloquine combinations used increasingly from 1991 and completely by 1994	Artesunate restores the cure rate; recrudescence rates are reduced and this lowers transmission
1995–99	Artesunate–mefloquine combination retains 100% efficacy after 4 years as first-line treatment; incidence of falciparum falls by 67% over the same period	Artesunate–mefloquine combination remains the treatment of choice in all camps in the area	Artesunate has prevented further selection of mefloquine resistance; its effect in reducing gametocyte carriage contributed to the fall in transmission

The experience in Karen refugee camps prompts the following conclusions:

- Applied and operational research on different drugs and regimens is the only way to develop a rational treatment policy in the face of increasing drug resistance.

- Simple, regular monitoring of drug resistance and a disciplined drug policy can prevent the development of drug resistance in refugee and non-refugee situations.

- In this area of low malaria transmission, early diagnosis and treatment with combined artesunate and mefloquine have reduced the incidence of *P. falciparum* malaria and halted the progression of mefloquine resistance.

Case Study 2. Prevention research (Kolaczinski et al., 2005)

Background

War, the breakdown of the health system, population displacement and poverty have led to a malaria epidemic in Afghanistan that has lasted for more than 20 years. The former, centrally managed, system of malaria control based on indoor spraying was no longer feasible or appropriate, and the only option possible in such unstable conditions was to help families to protect themselves. Questions related to the transformation from a system of total government provision to total self-reliance included:

- Which protection techniques are appropriate to the new conditions?

- Which delivery systems cover the most people at least cost?

- Who pays for the programme, and how much can beneficiaries contribute?

- What are the limitations of the strategy, what supplementary measures are needed to protect the poorest or to control malaria in the entire community?

A programme of operational research was needed to answer these questions, and in particular to:

- field-test potential control techniques in pilot projects;

- compare alternative delivery systems in terms of accessibility, coverage, and cost-effectiveness;

- field-test locally adapted information and promotional strategies designed to stimulate uptake.

Methods, results and lessons learned

Specific research studies were implemented at different stages to answer each of these questions, with research and control elements integrated in the same programme. As a result of this:

- A new kind of control programme evolved which emphasized protecting families by encouraging them to use ITNs, which had been shown to be locally effective.

- Treated nets were socially marketed through existing NGO clinics, private shops and pharmacies; this proved to be an efficient system that covered a high proportion of the population.

- Permethrin-treated top-sheets were promoted as a cheaper, but still effective, alternative for those unable to afford nets and for outbreak control.

The experience in Afghanistan prompts the following conclusions:

- Development of a malaria control programme is best guided by operational research.

- A series of fairly simple research questions and answers can lead to a culturally appropriate, effective, efficient and comprehensive prevention programme.

- Integration of operational research within a control programme generates a spirit of dynamism and prevents programme stagnation.

References

Bouma MJ et al. (1996). Malaria control using permethrin applied to tents of nomadic Afghan refugees in northern Pakistan. *Bulletin of the World Health Organization*, 74:413–421.

Chandre F et al. (1999). Current distribution of pyrethroid resistance gene (*kdr*) in *Anopheles gambiae* complex from West Africa and further evidence for reproductive isolation of the Mopti form. *Parasitologia*, 41: 319–322.

CIOMS (2002). *International ethical guidelines for biomedical research involving human subjects*. Geneva, Council for International Organizations of Medical Sciences.

Curtis CF et al. (1999). Malaria control: bednets or spraying? Summary of the presentations and the discussion. *Transactions of the Royal Society of Tropical Medicine and Hygiene*, 93:460.

Graham K et al. (2002). Insecticide-treated plastic tarpaulins for control of malaria vectors in refugee camps. *Medical and Veterinary Entomology*, 16:404–408.

Hargreaves K et al. (2000). *Anopheles funestus* resistant to pyrethroid insecticides in South Africa. *Medical and Veterinary Entomology*, 14: 181–189.

Kolaczinski JH et al. (2005). Subsidized sales of insecticide-treated nets in Afghan refugee camps demonstrate the feasibility of a transition from humanitarian aid towards sustainability. *Malaria Journal*, 3, 15.

Kolaczinski J et al. (2005). Malaria control in Afghanistan: progress and challenges. *Lancet*, 365:1506–1512.

Luxemburger C et al. (1994). Permethrin-impregnated bed nets for the prevention of malaria in schoolchildren on the Thai–Burmese border. *Transactions of the Royal Society of Tropical Medicine and Hygiene*, 88:155–159.

Nájera JA (1996). *Malaria control among refugees and displaced populations*. Geneva, World Health Organization (CTD/MAL/96.6).

Nosten F et al. (2000). Effects of artesunate-mefloquine combination on incidence of *Plasmodium falciparum* malaria and mefloquine resistance in western Thailand: a prospective study. *Lancet*, 356:297–302.

Pitt S et al. (1998). War in Tajikistan and re-emergence of *Plasmodium falciparum*. *Lancet*, 352:1279.

Rowland M (1999). Malaria control: bednets or spraying? Malaria control in the Afghan refugee camps of western Pakistan. *Transactions of the Royal Society of Tropical Medicine and Hygiene*, 93:458–459.

Rowland M, Hewitt S, Durrani N (1994). Prevalence of malaria in Afghan refugee villages in Pakistan sprayed with lambdacyhalothrin or malathion. *Transactions of the Royal Society of Tropical Medicine and Hygiene*, 88(4):378–379.

Rowland M et al. (1996). Pyrethroid-impregnated bed nets for personal protection from malaria for Afghan refugees. *Transactions of the Royal Society of Tropical Medicine and Hygiene*, 90:357–361.

Rowland M et al. (1997a). Sustainability of pyrethroid-impregnated bednets for malaria control in Afghan communities. *Bulletin of the World Health Organization*, 75:23–29.

Rowland M et al. (1997b). Resistance of falciparum malaria to chloroquine and sulfadoxine–pyrimethamine in Afghan refugee settlements in western Pakistan: surveys by the general health services using a simplified in vivo test. *Tropical Medicine and International Health*, 2:1049–1056.

Rowland M et al. (1999). Permethrin-treated chaddars and top-sheets: appropriate technology for protection against malaria in Afghanistan and other complex emergencies. *Transactions of the Royal Society of Tropical Medicine and Hygiene*, 93:465–472.

Rowland M et al. (2001). Control of malaria in Pakistan by applying deltamethrin insecticide to cattle: a community-randomised trial. *Lancet*, 357:1837–1841.

Rowland M et al. (2002a). Mosquito vectors and malaria transmission in eastern Afghanistan. *Transactions of the Royal Society of Tropical Medicine and Hygiene*, 96:620-626.

Rowland M et al. (2002b). Prevention of malaria in Afghanistan through social marketing of insecticide-treated nets: evaluation of coverage and effectiveness by cross-sectional surveys and passive surveillance. *Tropical Medicine and International Health*, 7:813–822.

Shah I et al. (1997). Chloroquine resistance in Pakistan and the upsurge of falciparum malaria in Pakistani and Afghan refugee populations. *Annals of Tropical Medicine and Parasitology*, 91:591–602.

Further reading

WHO (2000). *WHO Expert Committee on Malaria. Twentieth report.* Geneva, World Health Organization (WHO Technical Report Series, No. TRS 892).

- Has a useful chapter on operational research, available at www.who.int/malaria/docs/ecr20_9.htm.

WHO (2003). *Operational research for malaria control. Learner's guide and Tutor's guide* (trial edition). Geneva, World Health Organization, 2003 (WHO/HTM/RBM/2003.51 Part I and II).

- The *Learner's guide* covers basic concepts and information plus a series of problems, with hints or partial solutions to them. The document is available at http://www.who.int/malaria/docs/operational_research_lg.pdf.

Further information about operational research and ITNs can be found in:

- Chavasse D, Reed C, Attawell K (1999). *Insecticide-treated net projects: a handbook for managers.* London, Malaria Consortium.

Advice about field trials is available in:

- Smith PG, Morrow RH (1996). *Field trials of health interventions in developing countries – a toolbox.* London, Macmillan (see also Annex I).

Finding out more

The Malaria in Emergencies Network can provide technical assistance for the design, implementation and evaluation of operational research.

Malaria in Emergencies Network
World Health Organization
1211 Geneva 27
Switzerland
Fax: +41 22 791 4824
E-mail: rbmemergencies@who.int

Research assistance can also be obtained through the Malaria Consortium (www.malariaconsortium.org) or the London School of Hygiene & Tropical Medicine.

Mark Rowland
Department of Infectious Diseases
London School of Hygiene & Tropical Medicine
Keppel Street
London WC1E 7HT
England
Tel: +44 20 7299 4719
Fax: +44 20 7299 4720
E-mail: mark.rowland@lshtm.ac.uk

Annexes

Resources and web addresses

Note: The lists in this annex are provided for information only and should not be regarded as exhaustive, nor should the inclusion of any organization be construed as an endorsement.

Contributing agencies

Centers for Disease Control and Prevention
  www.cdc.gov

HealthNet International
  www.healthnetinternational.org

London School of Hygiene & Tropical Medicine
  www.lshtm.ac.uk

Malaria Consortium
  www.malariaconsortium.org

Médecins Sans Frontières (MSF)
  www.msf.org

Merlin
  www.merlin.org.uk

Office of the United Nations High Commissioner for Refugees (UNHCR)
  www.unhcr.ch

Shoklo Malaria Research Unit
  www.shoklo-unit.com

WHO Roll Back Malaria department
  www.who.int/malaria

United Nations and intergovernmental organizations

Department for Humanitarian Affairs (DHA)

Coordinates international emergency relief in complex emergencies.
  www.reliefweb.int

International Organization for Migration (IOM)

Intergovernmental organization, established in 1951 to resettle displaced European persons, refugees and migrants. Currently working with migrants and governments worldwide to provide humane responses to migration challenges.

www.iom.int

Office of the United Nations High Commissioner for Refugees (UNHCR)

Provides protection to refugees and seeks long-lasting solutions to their problems as well as providing essential materials and support in the country of refuge.

www.unhcr.ch

Roll Back Malaria (RBM) Partnership Secretariat

Ensures that contributions from individual RBM partners are coordinated and focused on the expressed needs of countries and in line with the best technical approaches. All activities are driven by the principal RBM objective – a rapid scaling-up of malaria interventions within countries, particularly to reach vulnerable populations.

www.rbm.who.int

United Nations Children's Fund (UNICEF)

Focuses on the needs of women and children in emergencies, including health, mental care, food, water and sanitation.

www.unicef.org

World Health Organization (WHO)

United Nations specialized agency for health.

www.who.int

- WHO Roll Back Malaria department
Web site: www.who.int /malaria
- WHO Health Action in Crises department
Web site: www.who.int/hac

World Food Programme (WFP)

Initiates and coordinates food aid for populations in acute emergencies through to rehabilitation and reconstruction phases.

www.wfp.org

United Nations Development Programme (UNDP)

Promotes measures for disaster prevention and mitigation and provides administrative support for United Nations Disaster Management Teams.
www.undp.org

United Nations Disaster Management Teams (UNDMT)

Normally chaired by the UNDP resident coordinator and includes representatives of all the above United Nations agencies. Aims to provide effective, coordinated United Nations response to support governments in emergencies.

Bilateral organizations

Australian Agency for International Development (AUSAID)
www.ausaid.gov.au

Department for International Development (DFID)
www.dfid.gov.uk

United States Agency for International Development (USAID)
www.usaid.gov

International foundations and associations

International Federation of Red Cross and Red Crescent Societies (IFRC)
www.ifrc.org

International Committee of the Red Cross (ICRC)
www.icrc.org

The Sphere Project
www.sphereproject.org

International Council of Voluntary Agencies
www.icva.ch

International NGOs and non-profit organizations

Africare
www.africare.org

Caritas International
www.caritas-international.de

Catholic Organisation for Relief and Development (CORDAID)
www.cordaid.nl

Epicentre
www.epicentre.msf.org

Food for the Hungry International
www.fh.org

Health Unlimited
www.healthunlimited.org

HealthNet International
www.healthnetinternational.org

International Centre for Migration and Health (ICMH)
www.icmh.ch

International Medical Corps
www.imcworldwide.org

International Rescue Committee (IRC)
www.theirc.org

Malaria Consortium
www.malariaconsortium.org

Médecins du Monde (MDM)
www.medecinsdumonde.org

Medair
www.medair.org

Mentor Initiative
www.mentor-initiative.net

Merlin
www.merlin.org.uk

Médecins Sans Frontières (MSF)
www.msf.org

Oxfam
www.oxfam.org.uk

Save the Children
www.savethechildren.org.uk

Trinity Health International
www.mercyinternational.com

US Committee for Refugees
www.refugees.org

Research & Development and Academic

Centers for Disease Control and Prevention
www.cdc.gov

London School of Hygiene & Tropical Medicine
www.lshtm.ac.uk

Johns Hopkins University
www.jhu.edu

Shoklo Malaria Research Unit
www.shoklo-unit.com

Regional NGO and Civil Societies

African Medical & Research Foundation (AMREF)
www.amref.org

Other organizations and resources

Amnesty International
www.amnesty.org

Center for Research on the Epidemiology of Disasters (CRED)
www.cred.be

Centro Regional de Informacion sobre Desastres (CRID)
www.crid.or.cr/crid

European Community Humanitarian Office (ECHO)
http://europa.eu.int/comm/echo

Mapping Malaria Risk in Africa
www.mara.org.za

Medline
www.ncbi.nlm.nih.gov/entrez/query.fcgi

Norwegian Refugee Council Global IDP Project
www.idpproject.org

Example consent form for surveys[1]

Location: .... Dwelling number: ....

We are from .... We are interested to know how much malaria there is in your community. Then we will know better how to stop people becoming sick and dying from malaria.

We would like to ask some questions and take a finger prick blood test (and examine you for signs of malaria[2]). The interview will take about .... minutes, and the blood test and examination will take .... minutes per person. If the blood test is positive for malaria, we will give you malaria treatment free of charge.

We cannot ask everyone in the community, so we are choosing some households at random. Your household has been selected. If you agree, we would like to ask you some questions, and to test you and everyone who normally sleeps in the house, including people who are not here right now, for malaria. We will do the test in your house at ....

Your participation is entirely voluntary. If you do not want to be part of this survey, you are free to say no. if you do not take part you are still welcome to come to the clinic for treatment, where services and treatment are free of charge.

Do you have any questions at this moment?

For more information and any questions on this survey, you can always contact ....

Thank you very much for participating in this survey.

Name: .... **Date:** ....

Signature: ....

Name of officer requesting consent: ....

---

[1] For more information: http://www.who.int/rpc/research_ethics/informed_consent/en/index.html.

[2] If temperature and spleen size are to be measured.

Worksheet: Rapid cross-sectional malaria prevalence survey

Malaria prevalence survey form   Date : _ _ / _ _ / _ _ _ _

Investigator's name:

Health zone:

Village:

Code _ _ _ _ _ _ _

Household number: _ _ _ _

Serial number	Sex		Age	History of fever during the past 48 hours?		Axillary temperature	Rapid test *P. falciparum* (RDT)		Treatment received in the past 7 days?		Where was treatment sought?								Treatment received?					Comments
	M	F	Years (<1 year = 0)	Yes	No	°C	+	–	Yes	No	hf	pf	m	ps	th	s	cq	sp	q	ACT	o	

Legend

hf: health facility   pf: private health facility   m: market   ps: private shop   th: traditional healers   s: personal stock

cq: chloroquine   sp: sulfadoxine–pyrimethamine   q: quinine   ACT: artemisinin-based combination therapy   o: other

Safety of antimalarial drugs for treatment and/or prophylaxis during pregnancy, breastfeeding and early childhood[1]

Note: Each drug also has its own side-effects and specific contraindications that should be taken into account.

Antimalarial drug	Indication	Pregnancy	Breast-feeding	Early childhood
Amodiaquine	Treatment	Apparently safe but limited data	No data	Safe
Artemether–lumefantrine	Treatment	Not recommended in 1st trimester because of lack of data	No data	Not recommended <5 kg because of lack of data
Artemisinin and derivatives	Treatment	Not recommended in 1st trimester because of lack of data	Safe	Safe
Atovaquone–proguanil	Prophylaxis Treatment	Very few data. Not recommended except as third-line "rescue" treatment for pregnant women with multidrug-resistant *P. falciparum* infection	No data, not recommended	Not recommended for prophylaxis in children <11 kg because of lack of data Apparently safe for treatment in children >5 kg, but limited data
Chloroquine	Prophylaxis Treatment (vivax only)	Safe	Safe	Safe
Clindamycin	Treatment (used in combination only)	Safe	Apparently safe but limited data	Apparently safe but limited data

[1] NB: No medication should be withheld if it is the only option available and would be life-saving in a laboratory-confirmed case of falciparum malaria.

Antimalarial drug	Indication	Pregnancy	Breast-feeding	Early childhood
Doxycycline	Prophylaxis (used alone) Treatment (used in combination only)	Contraindicated	Contra-indicated	Contraindicated <8 years of age
Mefloquine	Prophylaxis Treatment	Not recommended in 1st trimester because of lack of data	Safe	Not recommended <5 kg because of lack of data
Primaquine	Treatment	Contraindicated	Safe	Contraindicated <4 years of age
Proguanil	Prophylaxis (used in combination with chloroquine only)	Safe	Safe	Safe
Quinine	Treatment	Safe	Safe	Safe
Sulfadoxine–pyrimethamine	Treatment	Safe	Safe	Safe
Tetracycline	Treatment (used in combination only)	Contraindicated	Contra-indicated	Contraindicated <8 years of age

Dosage schedules for oral antimalarial drugs

For children, antimalarial drugs can be crushed, diluted in water and then either squirted directly into the mouth using a syringe or given with a spoon.

Artesunate + amodiaquine

This ACT is currently available only as separate scored tablets of artesunate (50 mg) and of amodiaquine (153 mg base). Co-formulated tablets are under development but are not yet available.

The recommended treatment is a once-daily dose of 4 mg/kg artesunate and 10 mg/kg amodiaquine base, given for 3 days.

Table A-V.1 **Dosage schedules for artesunate + amodiaquine**

Age	Artesunate tablets (50 mg)			Amodiaquine tablets (153 mg base)		
	Day 1	Day 2	Day 3	Day 1	Day 2	Day 3
5–11 months	$^1/_2$	$^1/_2$	$^1/_2$	$^1/_2$	$^1/_2$	$^1/_2$
≥1–6 years	1	1	1	1	1	1
≥7–13 years	2	2	2	2	2	2
≥14 years	4	4	4	4	4	4

Artemether–lumefantrine (Coartem®)

This ACT is currently available as co-formulated tablets each containing 20 mg of artemether and 120 mg of lumefantrine.

The recommended treatment is a 6-dose regimen containing 1.5 mg/kg artemether and 12 mg/kg lumefantrine twice daily for 3 days.

Table A-V.2 **Dosage schedules for artemether–lumefantrine (Coartem®)**

Weight (Approx. age)	No. of tablets at approx. timing (hours) of dosing					
	0 h	8 h	24 h	36 h	48 h	60 h
5–14.9 kg (<3 years)	1	1	1	1	1	1
15–24.9 kg (≥3–8 years)	2	2	2	2	2	2
25–34.9 kg (≥9–13 years)	3	3	3	3	3	3
>35 kg (≥14 years)	4	4	4	4	4	4

Simplification of the artemether–lumefantrine dosage schedule for ease of use at programme level is as follows:

— second dose on the first day to be given any time between 8 and 12 hours after the first dose;
— doses on the second and third days are given twice a day, morning and evening.

The 6-dose regimen of artemether–lumefantrine was previously not recommended for children weighing less than 10 kg. However, recent evidence suggests that therapeutic response and safety profile in young children are similar to those in older children, and the combination can now be given to children of body weight 5 kg and above.

Lumefantrine absorption is highly dependent on co-administration with fat. It is essential that patients or caregivers are informed of the need for artemether–lumefantrine to be taken with milk or other fat-containing food, particularly on the second and third days of treatment.

Artesunate + mefloquine

This ACT is currently available only as separate scored tablets of artesunate (50 mg) and of mefloquine (250 mg base). Co-formulated tablets are under development but are not yet available.

The recommended treatment is a once-daily dose of 4 mg/kg artesunate given for 3 days, combined with a total (split) dose of 25 mg/kg mefloquine base given either on the second (and third) day or in 3 days (8 mg/kg per day).

Table A-V.3 **Dosage schedules for artesunate + mefloquine**

Age	No. of artesunate tablets (50 mg) per day			No. of mefloquine tablets (250 mg base) per day		
	Day 1	Day 2	Day 3	Day 1	Day 2	Day 3
5–11 months	$^1/_2$	$^1/_2$	$^1/_2$	–	$^1/_2$	$^1/_2$
≥1–6 years	1	1	1	–	1	–
≥7–13 years	2	2	2	–	2	1
≥14 years	4	4	4	–	4	2

Vomiting is reduced if mefloquine is given on Day 2. If adherence is a problem, mefloquine can be given on Day 1.

Artesunate + sulfadoxine–pyrimethamine

This ACT is currently available only as separate scored tablets of artesunate (50 mg) and of pyrimethamine (25 mg) combined with sulfadoxine (500 mg). A similar formulation containing pyrimethamine (25 mg) combined with sulfalene (500 mg) is considered to be equivalent to sulfadoxine–pyrimethamine.

The recommended treatment is a once-daily dose of 4 mg/kg artesunate given for 3 days, combined with a single dose of sulfadoxine–pyrimethamine (25 mg/kg and 1.25 mg/kg) given on day 1.

Table A-V.4 **Dosage schedules artesunate + sulfadoxine–pyrimethamine (SP)**

Age	No. of artesunate tablets (50 mg) per day			No. of SP tablets (25 mg P + 500 mg S) per day		
	Day 1	Day 2	Day 3	Day 1	Day 2	Day 3
5–11 months	$^1/_2$	$^1/_2$	$^1/_2$	$^1/_2$	–	–
≥1–6 years	1	1	1	1	–	–
≥7–13 years	2	2	2	2	–	–
≥14 years	4	4	4	3	–	–

Although sulfadoxine–pyrimethamine is a single-dose treatment, artesunate must be given for 3 days to ensure satisfactory efficacy of the ACT.

Quinine

Oral quinine is available as scored tablets each containing either 200 mg or 300 mg quinine salt. Dosing with either formulation – 200 or 300 mg – leads to relative under- or overdosing at the extremes of the weight categories.

The recommended treatment is an 8-hourly (i.e. 3 times daily) dose of 10 mg/kg quinine salt given for 7 days.

Table A-V.5 **Dosage schedules for oral quinine**

If only the 200-mg quinine salt tablet is available:

Weight (kg)	No. of 200-mg tablets/dose
<8	$^1/_4$
8–12	$^1/_2$
13–17	$^3/_4$
18–25	1
26–35	$1^1/_2$
36–44	2
45–54	$2^1/_2$
≥55	3

If only the 300-mg quinine salt tablet is available:

Weight (kg)	No. of 300-mg tablets/dose
7–11	$^1/_4$
12–23	$^1/_2$
24–37	1
38–52	$1^1/_2$
≥53	2

If both 200-mg and 300-mg quinine salt tablets are available:

Weight (kg)	No. of 200-mg tablets/dose	No. of 300-mg tablets/dose
<8	$^1/_4$	–
8–12	$^1/_2$	–
13–17	$^3/_4$	–
18–23	1	–
24–37	–	1
38–52	–	$1^1/_2$
≥53	–	2

Chloroquine (for P. vivax only)

Chloroquine is available as scored tablets, usually containing either 100 mg or 150 mg chloroquine base per tablet. If formulations of other strengths are used, the dosage table below should be adjusted accordingly.

The recommended treatment is 25 mg/kg chloroquine base total, over 3 days. Chloroquine should be used only for the treatment of chloroquine-sensitive vivax malaria.

Table A-V.6 **Dosage schedules for chloroquine (for *P. vivax* only)**

Weight (kg)	Age	*either* No. of 100-mg tablets/day			*or* No. of 150-mg tablets/day		
		Day 1	Day 2	Day 3	Day 1	Day 2	Day 3
5–6	<4 months	$^1/_2$	$^1/_2$	$^1/_2$	$^1/_2$	$^1/_4$	$^1/_4$
7–10	4–11 months	1	1	$^1/_2$	$^1/_2$	$^1/_2$	$^1/_2$
11–14	1–2 years	$1^1/_2$	$1^1/_2$	$^1/_2$	1	1	$^1/_2$
15–18	3–4 years	2	2	$^1/_2$	1	1	1
19–24	5–7 years	$2^1/_2$	$2^1/_2$	1	$1^1/_2$	$1^1/_2$	1
25–35	8–10 years	$3^1/_2$	$3^1/_2$	2	$2^1/_2$	$2^1/_2$	1
36–50	11–13 years	5	5	$2^1/_2$	3	3	2
>50	≥14 years	6	6	3	4	4	2

Note: Chloroquine treatment for falciparum malaria is no longer acceptable for populations living in complex emergency situations. The only current exception to this rule is Haiti, where *P. falciparum* is known still to be fully sensitive to chloroquine.

Entomological investigations

This annex describes the basic methods used and the minimum information required for entomological investigations. More information about test methods is given in the following publications:

- WHO (1992). *Entomological field techniques for malaria control.* Part 1: Learners guide. Geneva, World Health Organization.
- WHO (1996). *Report of the WHO Informal Consultation on the evaluation and testing of insecticides, Geneva, 7–11 October 1996.* Geneva, World Health Organization (CTD/WHOPES/IC/96.1).

Surveillance

Before considerable resources are invested in specialized vector control programmes aimed at a reduction of malaria transmission, the following information is required:

- anopheline vector species present;
- relevant biology and behaviour (resting habits indoors and outdoors, feeding preferences, seasonal changes in abundance, locations found);
- breeding habits;
- resistance to insecticides.

The minimum information required is confirmation of vector species. Expertise in mosquito identification should be sought – locally if possible. Mosquitoes should be collected indoors and outdoors. The simplest method is indoor "fly spray" catches: exits are blocked off and mosquitoes are collected on floor sheets. Outdoors, mosquitoes can be collected using CDC light traps baited with CO_2 (dry ice) or by man-landing-catches using aspirators (sucking tubes). Knowledge of breeding habits is useful if breeding sites are limited and larviciding is feasible.

Resistance to insecticides

The standard method for detecting resistance is to expose mosquitoes to insecticide-treated papers within a WHO susceptibility test kit (obtain-

able from WHO – www.who.int/whopes/resistance/en/WHO_CDS_CPE_
PVC_2001.2.pdf). Field-collected mosquitoes are exposed to treated papers for 1 hour inside the kit, and the proportion killed is recorded after
a 24-hour recovery period. Resistance testing is especially important if
indoor residual spraying is being considered. Pyrethroid insecticides continue to work well in many regions but resistance is becoming increasingly
common in western and southern Africa.

Efficacy and residual life of insecticide treatments

Information on efficacy and residual life is needed if there is any doubt
about either the effectiveness of indoor spraying or the interval between
spray rounds. The simplest way of obtaining this information is by WHO
cone bioassay. A plastic cone is attached to the surface of sprayed walls.
Batches of field-caught mosquitoes are placed within the cone for 30 minutes, removed and transferred to a paper cup for observation; mortality is
determined after a 24-hour recovery period. Eight weeks after spraying, a
good insecticide should still give at least 70% mortality.

Householders who resent the intrusion of spray teams or object to spraying may re-plaster sprayed surfaces. There may be little that can be done to
counter this, but it would wise to monitor for evidence of re-plastering or
washing down of walls (using WHO cone bioassay tests, for example) to
guide future spraying policy.

It may be necessary to monitor the effectiveness of insecticide treatments
on nets. Most recommended pyrethroids give protection against mosquito
biting for at least 12 months after treatment. Marking nets with a non-per-
manent marker pen and then carrying out spot checks in the home provides
a means of monitoring washing rates. An alternative is to take samples of
netting and expose batches of mosquitoes to the treated surface using a
WHO cone bioassay test. If 50% of mosquitoes are knocked down after 10
minutes' exposure, the treatment can be considered to still be effective.

Questions to guide a rapid qualitative assessment of social, economic and cultural aspects of malaria

This annex is intended as a guide only: the questions that will need to be asked to understand what community members know about, and how they respond to, malaria will depend on the local situation and cultural norms. In addition, the approach used will depend on the subject group – key informants, householders, focus groups, etc. In some settings you may want to focus just on treatment-seeking behaviours or the use of preventive measures, while in other settings you may want a more complete understanding of what malaria means to a community and what they are most worried about. You can select the questions that you think are most relevant to what you need to know in order to make sound programmatic decisions related to malaria control in general. More information on preparing and carrying out social surveys is provided in the following publication:

* Akua Agyepong I et al. (1995). *The malaria manual – guidelines for the rapid assessment of social, economic, and cultural aspects of malaria.* Geneva, World Health Organization (TDR/SER/MRS/95.1).

Community perceptions of malaria

1. What are the common illnesses in the community?
   ➤ *Allow the person to list all illnesses, even if malaria or a malaria-like illness is not mentioned.*

2. Which of these illnesses are considered to be the most important?
   a) Why (prevalence, severity, mortality)?

3. Which of these illnesses affect children? Which affect adults?

4. What is the local name for "febrile illness"?
   ➤ *Probe for terms for febrile illness.*

5. Are there different types of febrile illness?
   a) If **yes**: What are the local names of these illnesses?
   b) Which of the febrile illnesses that you have described to me is considered to be the most dangerous?

c) How do you know when a child/an adult has this type of illness?

> *Identify which of the terms used for the illness most closely resembles the biomedical definition of malaria, then use that term for the questions below. In some cultures, fever with convulsions is considered to be a different type of malaria and one that is best suited for traditional or spiritual healing. If this is not mentioned, you could add a question such as "Is there a different illness when the child/adult has fever and also convulsions (shaking)?"*

6. What are the signs and symptoms of [local term for malaria]?

7. Who is most at risk for [local term for malaria]?

8. What causes [local term for malaria]?
   a) Can malaria be spread?
   b) If **yes**: How?
   > *If mosquitoes are not mentioned, probe with questions like: "Can this illness be carried by mosquitoes?"*

Treatment-seeking behaviours

9. How is [local term for malaria] treated?
   > *Probe to ensure that all treatments are mentioned, including use of self-medication.*
   a) Can you please tell me the steps of treatment once you notice that your child /an adult is sick with [malaria]?
   b) If **use of health care services** is mentioned: I see you mentioned going to the [dispensary/clinic/hospital] to receive care. From the time that you know that your child/the adult is sick, how long do you usually wait before going to the health care facility?
      —What do you do for treatment during times when the [dispensary/clinic/health post] might be closed (such as weekends, nights, holidays)?
      —Is there an ambulance service to help you with a really sick person?
      > *If the answer is **no**: probe to find out how they transfer a sick individual to a health care facility.*
   c) If **multiple treatments** are listed: do you use some of these treatments at the same time (for example, see a traditional healer for herbal treatments while taking antimalarials)?
   d) Which of these treatments are considered to be the most effective?
   e) From whom do you normally receive advice about how to treat illness in a child/adult?
   f) **If not previously mentioned**: Do you use the services of traditional healers or spiritualists for malaria?

212

—Do traditional healers ever give you antimalarial drugs?

g) Can you easily obtain drugs to treat [malaria] here in the camp/settlement area?

—If **yes**: where do you get these drugs?

h) Can you please tell me about any problems you might experience when seeking care from a health care facility in the camp/settlement area?

➤ *Probe for things such as lack of referrals, no assistance to transport a sick patient, long waiting periods for care, political/cultural differences with health care staff, perceived poor communication between staff and patients or caregivers, lack of drugs or other supplies.*

Prevention

10. Can [local term for malaria] be prevented?

a) If **yes**: How can you prevent it?

➤ *Probe for use of insecticides, bednets or other insecticide-treated materials, coils, repellents, etc.*

b) Of these methods, which ones do you personally use?

c) Why do you use these particular methods?

d) Which of the methods that you mentioned do you think are the most effective?

Insecticide-treated materials

11. In the residential unit that you live in, can you estimate for me how many households use insecticide-treated nets (ITNs)?

a) Would you say that your residential unit is similar to other parts of the camp/settlement area?

b) Did people bring the nets with them from their previous homes or did they receive them while they were in camp?

c) If a **net was mentioned** in response to question 10b): where and when did you get your net?

—Do you know whether your net was treated with insecticide?

—Have you ever had a net while in camp/settlement area that you needed to sell in order to buy more food?

—If the **interview is done at home** and if the respondent states that they have a net: Could you please show me your net?

➤ *Look to see what type of condition the net is in – is it dirty, is it very clean, does it have holes in it?*

d) If a **net was *not* mentioned** in response to question 10b): "I see that you did not mention using a bednet. Why is this?"

➤ *Probe for reasons of cost (cannot afford), lack of availability (such as distribution only to vulnerable populations), theft of nets, need to sell the net for food, dislike due to heat.*

e) Why do people use bednets?

➤ *Probe for prevention of nuisance biting, prevention of malaria, prestige, privacy.*

f) In your house, who sleeps under the net?

— Why does that person/those persons sleep under the net?

g) Are there any times when households in this area do not use nets if they have them?

➤ *Probe: "For example, what do people do when it is very hot outside? Do they sleep under the nets?"*

h) Do people always sleep indoors – or outside, or in fields?

i) Are nets supported by poles or are they suspended from ceilings?

j) What sizes and shapes of nets would best fit your sleeping arrangements?

Indoor residual spraying (IRS)

12. Have you ever had your house sprayed?

a) If **yes**: what did you think about that malaria control measure?

➤ *Probe: Ask whether they like the control measure; did they fear the insecticide being in the house.*

13. Do you think that this method works to control mosquitoes?

14. Was there anything that you did not like about IRS?

15. Once your house was sprayed, when did you next replaster the walls? (How much time elapsed between the spraying of the walls and replastering?)

Experience with malaria control

16. Did you have [local term for malaria] in your home area?

a) If **yes**: what was your experience with malaria control?

➤ *Probes: Ask whether they ever had indoor residual spraying done in their home; whether the health care facilities dispensed antimalarials; whether there were net distribution or insecticide re-treatment programmes taking place?*

b) Was the community involved in trying to control malaria?

— If **yes**: what did they do?

17. Can you please give me some ideas for what you would like to see in place in the camp to improve malaria control?

A checklist for effectively responding to malaria epidemics[1]

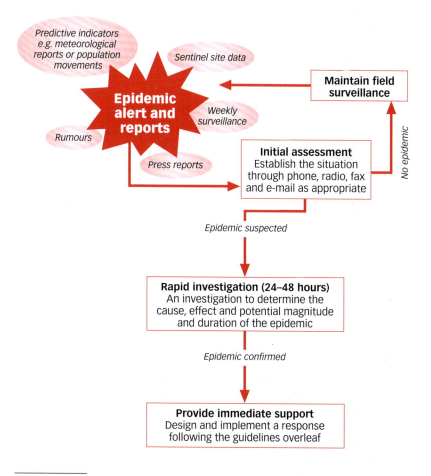

---

[1] Source: WHO (2002). *Prevention and control of malaria epidemics. Third meeting of the Technical Support Network.* Geneva, World Health Organization (WHO/CDS/RBM/2002.40): Annex 6 (with minor editorial changes).

Designing the response
At all epidemic stages

- Ensure that all clinics and health facilities are operational and have sufficient drugs, equipment and trained staff.
- Establish treatment centres (temporary clinics or mobile clinics) where access is a problem or health facility coverage is low.
- Ensure that the correct diagnosis and treatment is provided at all health facilities and at community level.
- Promote proactive clinical case detection and management/referral.
- Reinforce the referral system and consider the introduction of artesunate suppositories and IM artemether as a temporary measure where these are not already used.
- Intensify/maintain effective preventive measures for pregnant women.
- Reinforce health information systems for reporting and epidemic monitoring, preferably on a weekly basis.
- Conduct specific epidemic health education campaigns.
- Organize regular press releases/conferences/articles for public information.

Epidemic start

In the early stages of an epidemic, in addition to reinforcing case management (see above), it is still possible to reduce the potential impact of the epidemic using vector control interventions such as indoor residual spraying (IRS).

Additional specific interventions

- *If the area is in principle already protected by IRS* – establish coverage and quality of vector control using techniques such as bioassays.
- *If the area is not already protected*, but the malaria epidemiology, type of housing and available logistics allow rapid deployment of effective IRS – implement IRS in target areas.

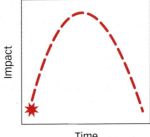

- *Consider* – properly timed fogging in highly populated areas such as refugee/displaced persons camps, especially if shelters are small and IRS is not an option.
- *Consider* – re-impregnation or use of ITMs (insecticide-treated materi-

als including bednets) if there is a history of ITM use in the area or if the capacity exists to enforce such a programme (e.g. within a concentrated workforce).

Epidemic acceleration

Case management (see above) is the priority at this stage. Aiming to reduce the potential impact of the epidemic through IRS and other vector control methods is an option only if (1) there is considerable operational capacity trained and readily available, and (2) preparedness levels have been high.

Additional specific interventions

- *Consider* – establishing coverage and quality of vector control, using techniques such as bioassays, if the area has already been sprayed.
- *Consider* – IRS if the area is not already protected.
- *Consider* – changing chemicals for IRS if observed susceptibility is low.
- *Consider* – properly timed fogging in highly populated areas such as refugee/displaced persons camps, especially if shelters are small and IRS is not an option.

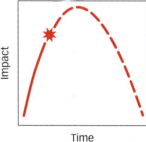

Epidemic peak

The epidemic has already begun to stabilize at this point and the number of new cases is beginning to decrease. Vector control interventions to reduce the potential impact of the epidemic have no public health value at this late stage. Resources should instead be directed at case management to reduce malaria mortality (see above).

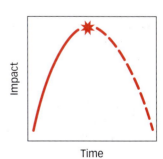

After epidemics

Ensure lessons-learned exercise ("postmortem") for next epidemic.

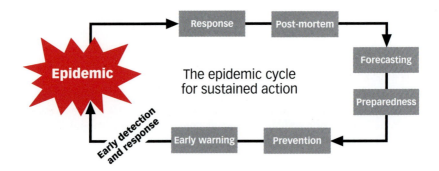

The epidemic cycle for sustained action

Pre-season preparedness and early identification provide the malaria manager with an increasing number of tools to deal with an epidemic. Maintain surveillance, keep database up to date, think ahead – **be prepared**.